The Irving B. Harri{
of the ZERO TO TH

Kadija Johnson and Charles Brinamen are the winners of a 2003 Irving B. Harris Award of the ZERO TO THREE Press. Created by the late Irving B. Harris, these generous stipends offered essential support to outstanding authors for the development of book manuscripts that address issues of emerging importance to the multidisciplinary infant–family field. The ZERO TO THREE Press Editorial Board selected the recipients from among manuscripts submitted for consideration during five competitions in 2003 through 2005. *Mental Health Consultation in Child Care: Transforming Relationships Among Directors, Staff, and Families* is in large measure a result of Harris' generosity and belief in the power of books to make a lasting difference in the way we care for infants, toddlers, and families.

MENTAL HEALTH CONSULTATION IN CHILD CARE

Transforming Relationships Among Directors, Staff, and Families

KADIJA JOHNSTON
AND **CHARLES BRINAMEN**

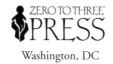

ZERO TO THREE
PRESS

Washington, DC

Published by

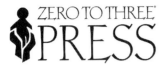

ZERO TO THREE
2000 M St., NW, Suite 200
Washington, DC 20036-3307
(202) 638-1144
Toll-free orders (800) 899-4301
Fax: (202) 638-0851
Web: http://www.zerotothree.org

The mission of the ZERO TO THREE Press is to publish authoritative research, practical resources, and new ideas for those who work with and care about infants, toddlers, and their families. Books are selected for publication by an independent Editorial Board.
The views contained in this book are those of the authors and do not necessarily reflect those of ZERO TO THREE: National Center for Infants, Toddlers and Families, Inc.

Cover design: Jennifer Paul
Text design and composition: Design Consultants, Inc.

Library of Congress Cataloging-in-Publication Data

Johnston, Kadija.
    Mental health consultation in child care : transforming relationships among directors, staff, and families / Kadija Johnston & Charles Brinamen.
        p. cm.
    Includes bibliographical references.
    ISBN-13: 978-0-943657-91-2
    ISBN-10: 0-943657-91-1
    1. Child mental health services. 2. Day care centers—Psychological aspects. I. Brinamen, Charles. II. Title.
    [DNLM: 1. Mental Health Services. 2. Child Care—psychology.
    3. Child Day Care Centers. 4. Referral and Consultation. 5. Infant.
    6. Child, Preschool.   WS 105.5.M3 J72m 206]
RJ499.J565 2006
618.92'89—dc22   2006003352

10 9 8 7 6 5 4 3 2 1
ISBN 0-943657-91-1
Printed in the United States of America

Suggested citation:
Johnston, K., & Brinamen, C. (2006). *Mental health consultation in child care: Transforming relationships among directors, staff, and families.* Washington, DC: ZERO TO THREE Press.

Dedication

To my dear papa.
You knew it would be and it was. My gratitude for your guidance. – KJ

To my grandmother. – CFB

Table of Contents

Foreword

This is a wonderful book. It is intelligent, thoughtful, and engaging; it stems from nearly 20 years of continuous, examined provision of mental health consultation to a wide range of settings and communities. Daycare Consultants' approach to mental health consultation is a way of learning that relies on collaboration at every hand. It also relies on respect, flexibility, self-examination, openness to the other, and a willingness to examine assumptions and imagine their opposites. This approach demands the capacity to hold contradictory ideas in mind. It treasures uncertainty and attentive, inclusive interaction. It necessitates remembering the power of role and appreciates empathy and reality as the attitudinal underpinnings of curiosity. Skills and knowledge can only be successfully actualized in this context. These are some of the overarching messages of this book.

Daycare Consultants: History and Influences

No service program is without a significant history or conflux of influences. Many people, events, and ideas are represented in the form and directions a program takes as it begins, and as it evolves. Daycare Consultants grew out of the Infant–Parent Program (IPP), which was established at the University of California, San Francisco in 1979. IPP, in turn, was a flexible transplant of Selma Fraiberg's Child Development Project at the University of Michigan. Her innovative brand of "kitchen-table" infant–parent psychotherapy took root and flourished during the 1970's. When, a decade later, IPP therapists realized that infant–toddler staff in child-care centers could benefit from support as much as parents, they used IPP's ways of approaching and understanding human beings to create Daycare Consultants. Both programs bear the imprint of the breadth and sensibilities of the world of social work and the more internal focus of the psychodynamic world as well. Ms. Fraiberg herself was a vibrant embodiment of both perspectives.

A second influence on Daycare Consultants was the National Center for Clinical Infant Programs, the organization that is now known as ZERO TO THREE. Selma Fraiberg was one of the founders of this group, which from its inception worked to acknowledge and integrate the knowledge and perspectives of its members' highly developed areas of expertise; such integration was, in fact, its reason for being. This passionate group of pioneers was in love with babies— their beginnings and their wondrous possibilities for development. They cared deeply about understanding the nurturing roles of those privileged to care for them.

The founders of ZERO TO THREE loved learning about infants, toddlers, and their families from one another. Over the years, both the IPP mutual exchange of knowledge and Daycare Consultants benefited from ZERO TO THREE's model of considering mutual exchange of knowledge an absolute necessity for research and practice in the infant–family field. Endorsing this principle ensured that Daycare Consultants would be devoted to learning from others at every level— each center and family child-care home and each of their diverse larger communities. They would learn, as well, from other community professionals, and everyone encountered in their direct clinical work. Daycare Consultants brought this perspective into the world of child care.

Fraiberg' seminal Child Development Project demanded that its dedicated practitioners gather regularly around a table to clarify what they were doing with infants and families, and why. Daycare Consultants established the same process at its beginning and maintained it throughout its growth. The program's staff discussions were characterized by care, deliberation, and sometimes insight and inspiration.

Goodness of fit between infant–parent psychotherapy and consultation to child care became apparent when the IPP made contact with Early Childhood Mental Health, a nonprofit agency, in Contra Costa County. We helped them add an Infant–Parent Program to their existing therapeutic nursery school. The nursery school's director, Lenore Thompson, subsequently began a consultation program to child-care settings, using teams of social workers and early childhood educators. Representatives of IPP were involved in consulting.

Within this context and through the good offices of child development expert and philanthropist Marilyn Segal and the generosity of the Stuart Foundation, Daycare Consultants was launched in 1988 as a component of IPP. The first decisions involved how and where the services should be delivered, who the consultants should be, and whether the services should be city-wide or limited to specific sites. The decision was to cast the widest net possible and to include all centers and family child-care homes, no matter their sources of support. Consultants' visits would be on site and open-ended, and would continue on a mutually determined basis. Potential consultants would be considered on the basis of their knowledge and experience with infants, toddlers, and preschoolers, and their knowledge and experience in the mental health field. Interviewers would look for evidence of cultural intelligence, open-mindedness, and appreciation of the needs of parents, teachers, and children. They would also work to make sure that the group of consultants would represent the varied communities and languages of the city.

The group had to decide how to introduce themselves to the child-care community. Daycare Consultants wanted to invite, but not solicit, community child-care programs to use their new service. They wanted to make it clear that programs were not expected to know in advance all that they might need from a mental health consultant. The child-care program and Daycare Consultants would determine together what each center or family child-care home wished to pursue. Each of the programs would contribute to the overall evolution of the service.

Mental Health Consultation to Child Care: Learning From Everyone

In *Mental Health Consultation in Child Care: Transforming Relationships Among Directors, Staff, and Families*, Kadija Johnston and Charles Brinamen demonstrate again and again how collaboration, respect, flexibility, self-examination, openness, tolerance for ambiguity, and a commitment to understanding everyone's perspective can transform relationships and, thereby, young children's experience in child care. The authors describe in detail how the process of transformation begins and continues with everyone the consultants encounter. They recognize that understanding the relationships that are being engendered by all the people in the child-care setting—including the consultant—is central to ultimate understanding of the experiences of children, parents, and caregivers.

The authors show how consultants make the effort to understand again and again, in different guises, with everyone they encounter. They also demonstrate the mental health consultant's need for basic knowledge of child and adult development, group process, and the dynamics of interpersonal relationships. Just as one searches to begin to understand the meaning of a child's behaviors in the "now," one does the same for the teacher, parent, grandmother, bus driver, and director. The consultant is open to learning equally from all of them what they are experiencing. This is never a game in which someone either wins or is a loser. It is real life. Striving for inclusiveness and collaboration and avoiding premature closure is the promising, if bumpy, road to success.

All of us can learn to be smart about people, and we need to be, but we need to remember that each person is the final confirmation of herself and what she feels. These authors never abandon this insight. They remind us that the smallest infant can tell us much about himself if we look long and listen well before we cross the boundary between pondering and possibly knowing.

Registering and Evaluating Experience

One of the greatest virtues of this book is its ability to capture the complexities of the consultant's internal processes as she registers her experience and evaluates it. The consultant is striving simultaneously to apprehend and examine the experience of others; she melds each new insight with her experience, knowledge, and developing understanding of the context in which she is working. She applies her enriched awareness to each individual involved in the consultation process, and to their interactions. Everyone with whom the consultant interacts should feel seen, heard, and, as much as possible, understood.

The consultant's task is truly a matter of internal and external juggling. But the juggling metaphor should not at all suggest neglect of any of the balls in the air, but rather the effort required to keep any of the balls from hitting the floor— at least not very often. The consultant must also strive to hold a calm center as a necessary internal state. As the authors demonstrate, achieving and maintaining calm is not always easy. Success depends not only on skill and expertise but also on the consultant's firm belief in the utter necessity of a calm center. Maintaining it relies on an awareness of what is and what is not one's responsibility, and what is or is not in one's ability to control. As *Mental Health Consultation in Child Care* asserts and demonstrates, the foremost professional responsibility of anyone in the child-care environment is to be aware of one's own feelings and the impact of one's own actions and meaning on another, in ways both obvious and subtle. Human communication occurs along every avenue of expressiveness, unintentionally and intentionally. The vivid material in this book presents many views of this professional use of self.

The intensity of focus and process in mental health consultation to child care engage so much of a consultant's personhood that the work is exhilarating as well as demanding. Yet the calm center that allows hyperalertness and delicate sensitivity does not at all require hair-trigger action. On the contrary, it prevents it.

Both the narrative sections and the many vignettes in this book articulate the consultant's experience as observer, interpreter, and participant. The authors' presentation of rapid, internal, in-the-moment processes allows the reader to glimpse inside the consultant as she experiences the kaleidoscope of activity and human connection and disconnection, actual and psychological. The activities of children and staff are a free-form ballet that, if speeded up, would make anyone grin. But the authors slow down the tempo of the dance when they turn to the consultant's process. Doing so allows the reader a deep appreciation for the feelings alive in the classroom or staff room, and for those alive in the consultant. All are interesting, compelling, and important. Everyone's feelings potentially lead in different directions. The careful articulation of the consultant's internal experience, the processing of a multitude of considerations, constructions, simultaneous possibilities, and, then, an eventual expressed communication is continuously illuminating.

Paradoxically, the time it takes to read accounts of what the consultant is experiencing and processing helps the reader appreciate the actual rapidity of the steps that make up the consultative process. One realizes, for example, that a page-long account of an interaction with a child represents what is in reality a split-second of complex, affective thinking. Only upon reflection and self-examination can the consultant can become truly aware of all she observed, thought, and acted upon in the moment. The reader learns more. As the authors describe both the breadth and the challenge of multi-attentional observation and processing, they identify what needs to occur, often in concrete examples. Should the consultant ask a question of Tamara, turn to Fred and make eye contact, express her puzzlement, make a suggestion or an observation, or simply wait with interest? These are lightning-speed decisions, but never unconsidered. The authors consistently illustrate what the consultant needs to be apprehending and processing in order to be effective. Obviously, as we practice our skills, many sequences of observation, reflection, interpretation, and response become more automatic as they come to "live in our bones." Still, every encounter with a child or adult is new. Each one calls for fresh and continuous awareness.

Descriptions of the consultant at work in the child-care setting make the consultant's need for reflective supervision abundantly clear. The authors have made the inspired choice to follow each description of a consultant's work with a description of a meeting between the consultant and her supervisor. In their relationship to the consultants, the (fictionalized) supervisors embody the same qualities of consideration, understanding, questioning, and openness that the consultants are learning to master.

Many of the vignettes in this book manage to illustrate vividly and concretely such abstract concepts as: levels of mutually influencing practices; conflicting attitudes among institutions, practitioners, directors, parents, children, and communities; and the hierarchical standing of various entities and people. Again and again, the authors point out pathways through these thickets of human interaction, influence, and power. A reader might fear being overwhelmed by this book's comprehensive treatment of the large issues involved in mental health consultation in child care and its equally detailed exploration of individual elements of the work. Such a fear is not entirely irrational. However, this book is eminently practical. The authors consistently suggest a multitude of possibilities for understanding situations, potential avenues for intervention, and a way of finding the next step.

A glance at the chapters and their contents will assure anyone that the authors leave no stone unturned or unexamined in the child-care playground. A few stones are occasionally flung—most signally at power brokers who fail to recognize the importance of excellent child care to the mutual care and raising of children by parents and their communities.

Spirals of influence

The authors of *Mental Health Consultation in Child Care* consider every role in the child-care environment. This book is truly inclusive. It is also generous to and respectful of human beings and their challenges.

There is expertise and there is storytelling in this book. Some stories continue across chapters, like movie serials or what-is-next soap operas. These tales are reliably enlivening as well as illuminating.

As one reads this book, one realizes that it follows a course of expanding spirals of influence. Each story recounts the experience of a child, but the spheres of influence that each child inhabits are all recognized. They are both generic (e.g., the foster care system) and specific (e.g., the grudge match between two teachers in a child-care classroom). The consultant is shown trying to understand and respond to these elements in a thoughtful, planful, and inclusive way, in a natural flow from each child. Because the consultants realize that they cannot learn by guessing what someone feels or thinks, they wait, wonder, listen, and collaborate. Everyone must be considered, seen, and heard. Everyone must feel considered, seen, and heard.

Why You Will Be Extremely Happy That You Own This Book

This book should be widely appreciated. It will surely capture the full attention of the growing number of agencies and individual practitioners who are embarking on mental health consultation in child care or are preparing to do so. The authors offer consultants with some experience an organized framework for considering the complexities of their work and an abundance of insights and ideas to enrich their practice. Practitioners, supervisors, teachers, and students in early care and education, the mental health professions, family support, and all disciplines concerned with the development of young children will benefit from a journey through this book.

Young children, with their individual strengths and needs, are surrounded by worlds of influence that affect their experience. Those in a position to affect those influences, whether individuals or institutions, need to be aware of their power and determined to use it positively. Children deserve our strongest possible efforts on their behalf. How children's possibilities emerge and can be realized depends in significant measure on the contributions of those who directly care for them—including, surely, the child-care community. This book has a great deal to add to our national conversation about how to strengthen the people and the relationships that shape the daily care of our young children. *Mental Health Consultation in Child Care* is a needed, valuable, and most welcome contribution.

Jeree H. Pawl, PhD
Mill Valley, California

Acknowledgments

It is with profound gratitude that we acknowledge the people whose energy and effort permeate these pages.

Developing and describing the approach to consultation in this book depended on the immense skill, dedication, and talent of many colleagues and numerous supporters. We have had the privilege of pondering the tiny triumphs and daily dilemmas of consultation with a truly amazing and unique cohort (Abby, Adriana, Amee, Betsy B., Betsy W., Cheryl, Cynthia, Donna W., Elea, Elizabeth, Farris, German, Hector, Isela, Jennifer, Jeree, Judy, Kim, Kristin, Laurel, Lea, Leslie, Liz, Maria, Mariam, Melissa, Michele, Miriam, Rita, Sandra). Their collective wisdom challenged us to capture the complexity of our consultative efforts and sustained us in doing so. Child-care providers, directors, and families permitted us to share in and learn from their struggles and strivings on behalf of young children.

We are indebted to our funders. The Stuart Foundation embraced an idea. Amy Rassen of Jewish Family and Children's Services, Sai-Ling Chan Sew of San Francisco's Community Behavioral Health Services/Department of Public Health, the Miriam and Peter Haas Foundation, the San Francisco Department of Human Services and First Five San Francisco took up the torch and turned a vision into an established network of support.

Blanca's boundless energy and generosity and Pilar's steady spirit of support made the undoable effortless, crises ephemeral, and the elusive tangible.

We are grateful for the guidance of Emily Fenichel, our inspired and inspiring editor who polished our prose, and to Jennifer Moon and the rest of the ZERO TO THREE Press team for finessing the final product.

Kadija

With immeasurable appreciation and love, I want to express my gratitude:

To my parents, Jim and Rosa, for bringing me into being. They, along with my beloved sister Deidre, Wayne, Johnston, and Ellis accompany and applaud each step of my becoming. To my soul twin Brian for encouraging, admiring, and envisioning with an unwavering assurance that made this and all my imaginings possible. To the rest of my soul cluster, Pam, Heff, and Terri—our entwined existence and evolution brought me to and carried me through the big wave. To my mentors and other mothers, Jeree and Lenore, who saw the spark, ignited passion, and blazed the trail. It is an honor to follow in the path lit by your brilliance. To my co-author Charles, whose clarity and calm made co-creating meaning a lively lived experience. To Laurel, my conspirator in proliferating a vision and partner in the transcendent power of practice.

Charles

Consultation, like life and this book, is foremost a collaborative effort. The people who have helped me to become, to be, and to work fill these pages. I am truly grateful for their contributions. Farris Page, my mentor and friend, invited me to share in her consultation efforts. She has been generous with her time, thoughts, spirit, and laughter. The Children's Council, especially its Executive Director Linnea Klee, introduced me to Farris and this work and allowed me to follow my interests. It was through these experiences that I came to know Kadija, who shared her insights and helped me to shape my own. Collaborating with her has been an exciting, stimulating endeavor. My work is deeper and richer for knowing her. I am also indebted to David R., who helped me find my voice. Val taught me to put my thoughts on paper (and edit, edit, edit).

I have been lucky to have the love and support of generous family and friends with diverse talents. For over a year, Lee welcomed me back from writing weekends and evenings away with love and support, making this process easier. I am grateful for his steady contribution. Roz helps me to find humor in the frustrating, allowing me to return to life and work with renewed energy. Robert, who challenges me to think more deeply, introduced me to the book that inspired the vignette format that leaps from chapter to chapter. Dona's probing, detailed questions help me to live honestly. I am thankful for these and other friends who tolerated my absences and continued to offer warmth and understanding. They remained interested and excited for me even when my own resolve waned. Some others should also be mentioned by name: David, Dora, John, Lovely and Jassi, Micki, Natasha and Sean, and Rachelle.

My sister Maribeth, who has given birth to a small family child care, including two twin studies, makes me laugh, offers support, and shares her experiences of typically developing children—excuse me, *above* averagely developing children. Matthew, Christopher, Patrick, William, Jacob, and Andrew regularly make me smile and appreciate life, teach me about the complexity of nature and nurture, and remind me why this work is so important. Their father, Greg, is always big-hearted.

My mother was already "thinking together" about child care and children with special needs when I was a child. Her work anticipated this work. Finally, I am grateful for the love of caring, accepting parents. I hope that I bring their same generosity of spirit to consultation and to these pages.

Introduction

Babies are inherently social beings. The quality of their primary relationships largely determines their sense of self and indeed the whole course of their development. Through interactions with parents and other caregivers, a baby learns about the world—what it feels like, smells like, and tastes like; what can be expected; what can be controlled; how responsive it is; and how harsh or benign. The experience that a child accumulates in the earliest years of life becomes a continuous, organizing filter for all subsequent experience.

For many babies, toddlers, and preschoolers, much of their experience takes place in child care. Thus the quality of relationships between caregivers and children (and, as we shall see, the quality of caregiver–parent and caregiver–colleague relationships) affects every child in the child-care setting. More specifically, the impact and quality of caregivers' relationships with children contribute to the quality of young children's mental health. When very young children are in distress, child-care providers face many of the same challenges as parents in understanding and caring for them. This is especially true when a child's relationships have been or continue to be troubled.

A mental health consultant who understands the development of young children, the experiences of parents, and the world of child care can help to strengthen or, if need be, repair relationships in a child-care setting. Because the quality of caregiver–child relationships is affected by the adult's history and capacity for relationships, the mental health consultant considers and attends to the needs of adults as often as to the needs of children. Services range from case consultation, which addresses the needs of individual children, to program consultation, which explores a range of circumstances in the child-care setting. Mental health consultants look at the way that caregivers engage each other, the context in which staff relationships evolve, the training of providers, the idiosyncrasies and individual needs of the caregiving adults, and each program's uniquely enacted philosophy, functioning, and history.

Mental health consultation to child care is not a new phenomenon but is expanding from the circumscribed approach of the 1950s, which focused on a single child, to include the system of child care. As the number of children and the hours they participate in child care increase exponentially (with the most dramatic increases occurring in infant care), the demands and reliance on child care are overtaxing child care and its providers. The quality of care is more important now than ever because children's development largely occurs in the context of child care. Unfortunately, the quality has not kept up with the demand.

We know that quality care, necessary for a child's healthy development and dependent on the adult–child and, therefore, adult relationships, is most highly correlated with staff wages. In fact, most indicators of quality begin with adult characteristics: staff pay, training, and longevity. Ratio and group size, other important predictors of quality, are also linked with the adults' experience and the money available for child care. In a field that is undervalued, the dollars devoted to these measures of quality are limited. We can infer that provider–child relationships are suffering, and those that can least afford it are suffering most.

In addition, more and more children are entering child care with challenges associated with poverty, violence, drug use, and their effects on individuals and the community. Increasingly, those concerned about vulnerable children are turning to child care to ameliorate the consequences of deprivation and loss and to reverse challenging behaviors—all this at a time when child-care providers have increased dramatically in number but typically lack enough training or experience to support these extra responsibilities. Because more families depend on child care, whether by circumstance or choice, more children who may not temperamentally fit the child-care setting are shoe-horned into care.

Regardless of etiology or the age at which a child's difficulties are discovered, child-care programs are struggling to respond to the growing number of children with puzzling developmental profiles and challenging behaviors. Caregivers report that more children with greater emotional and developmental difficulties are entering their programs each year (Yoshikawa & Knitzer, 1997) and that they do not feel equipped to deal with these special needs (Knitzer, 1996). Even when providers are intellectually equipped to understand and respond to children with difficulties, the distress that a child's troubling behavior demonstrates can be overwhelming.

Responding in an environment of overwhelming demands (both in numbers and quality of need) with decreasing resources, the mental health consultant has a daunting—and often lonely—job. Ideally, case conferences and supervision offer consultants opportunities for support, reduce isolation, and propose alternative explanations and ideas. We hope that this book will serve a similar function for prospective or beginning mental health consultants, more seasoned consultants who are feeling stuck or alone, and programs or agencies that are considering mental health consultation as a way of strengthening their early childhood systems of care.

This guide is the outgrowth of the authors' experiences in founding and working in Daycare Consultants, which is an extension of the Infant–Parent Program of the University of California, San Francisco, a program that provides treatment to troubled parent–child relationships. Before coming to the Infant–Parent Program, the authors developed ideas about consultation by working with others who provided similar services to child care: Lenore Thompson of the Early Childhood Mental Health Program and Farris Page of the Children's Council of San Francisco. These experiences contributed to the current conceptualization of consultation honed at Daycare Consultants. A brief history of Daycare Consultants may be the best way to introduce the approach to mental health consultation described in this book.

The History of Daycare Consultants

In 1979, Selma Fraiberg and her colleagues came from Ann Arbor, Michigan, to the University of California, San Francisco to begin the Infant–Parent Program. Fraiberg brought with her ideas and experiences about effecting change in troubled relationships that were based on her earlier work with blind infants and their parents. She was convinced that exploration of a parent's feelings and disappointments, combined with developmental guidance, could transform parent–child relationships and, therefore, a child's development. By addressing these relationships, a therapist could effect positive change in an infant's development and experience in the world.

Recognizing that impediments to healthy development extend beyond congenital limitations such as blindness, Fraiberg and her colleagues applied their intervention to other at-risk infant populations. Combining principles from the fields of social work and psychoanalysis, they visited parents in their homes to understand the rhythms of and to make an impact within the child and parents' real routines and to ensure contact with parents who were too overwhelmed to visit a therapist's office. Through these experiences, Fraiberg and her colleagues identified what they called "the ghosts in the nursery." These were mothers' painful memories of their own childhoods, which interfered with their ability to respond sensitively to their children. With thoughtful and compassionate consideration of the mothers' experience, the "kitchen-table" therapists worked to liberate the infants from the hostile hold of the parents' past. If a baby had constitutional challenges, making it more difficult to care for him, the infant–parent psychotherapists offered empathy for the parent's pain, tried to create understanding of the child's contribution and experience, and offered caregiving ideas that might make interaction easier for both. Always they aimed to improve the parent–child relationship.

The Development of Daycare Consultants

In 1988, the Infant–Parent Program established Daycare Consultants. In doing so, the program extended its philosophy of treating young children in the context of defining relationships to child care. At this time, infant–toddler child care was becoming more and more prominent in the Infant–Parent Program's direct clinical work—in part because child care was becoming more widely used in the community. Sometimes, Infant–Parent Program therapists looked to child care as a respite for a distressed parent and an intervention for the child in the hope that positive child–caregiver interactions might constitute a corrective emotional experience. But as program psychotherapists came in contact with child-care providers more frequently, they realized that child-care providers had many of the same challenges as parents, especially with children whose relationship histories were worrisome. Because the quality of caregiver–child relationships clearly affected all of the children in a program, Daycare Consultants was conceived in order to address the impact of these relationships on *all* children in the setting not only those who had been identified as in distress.

Funding for Daycare Consultants came initially from private foundations. Later, when the public became aware of child care's increasing woes and responsibilities, money became available through various departments of the City and County of San Francisco. In 1994, these grants led to collaboration with other institutions that were beginning to provide mental health consultation to child care. This proliferation encouraged community-wide support, which, in turn, led to more programs providing mental health consultation in the City. Now, any child-care program (center or family child care) in the city or county of San Francisco that wishes to have mental health consultation can do so.

Since 1996, Daycare Consultants has trained and supervised mental health consultants who are employed by Jewish Family and Children's Services of the Bay Area. Between the two programs, at least 15 consultants provide services across several Bay Area Counties. In addition, each year a group of trainees is learning and practicing the specifics of mental health consultation to child care.

Daycare Consultants' Training and Supervision

Mental health consultation requires such a broad knowledge base that no one person could possibly have experience in all aspects of the work. A competent mental health consultant needs to understand principles underlying early childhood education, child development, and mental health. Most would-be consultants have experience in one area or another but need training to fill in gaps in their expertise. Clinicians need to familiarize themselves with the complexities of group care and make distinctions between consultation and treatment. Because mental health professionals are trained to focus on pathology, they may need to refresh or expand their knowledge of typical development. Because most issues that program consultation covers concern adult interaction and organizational functioning, new consultants need to understand group work with adults and systems.

No consultant begins with all of the expertise needed for her job. We have found, however, that focusing on specific content areas and cultivating a particular perspective make the task of mastering the knowledge base less formidable. These areas are as follows:

1. *Self-awareness.* Consultants must be able to observe themselves and to identify their own feelings, biases, and impact on others.

2. *Knowledge of infant mental health principles.* Direct experience with young children brings the fullest and deepest understanding of these principles, which help the consultant understand the child's perspective. Understanding the mutually influencing system of infant and caregiver assists consultants in sorting out difficulties in those relationships.

3. *Experience working with parents.* Work with the parents of young children prepares consultants to address parents' normal fears, projections, and misunderstandings. Such experience makes it easier to maintain a neutral and receptive stance in the face of problematic parenting practices.

4. *Familiarity with typical child development.* Knowledge of typical child development in all its complexity helps the mental health consultant consider multiple contributors to a child's developmental status and sort out the various causes of a child's challenges. The consultant can use her knowledge of typical development to reduce caregivers' tendency to blame the child for behavioral shortcomings and to align expectations to a child's abilities.

5. *Group facilitation skills.* A large component of the work of consultation is interacting with and facilitating groups of teachers. Child-care professionals have varying levels of education, experiences, and cultural constructions about caring for children, and, therefore, often have difficulty communicating with each other. The consultant is called on to interpret each individual's unique perspective to the others in an effort to assist in developing a unified approach to their work with children.

6. *Appreciation of group care.* A successful consultant, even when addressing concerns about a particular child, must take into consideration the constraints of group care—both other children's reactions as well as the caregivers' abilities to meet the needs of an individual within the context of the group setting.

7. *Curiosity and respect for differences.* Our relational work requires respect for cultural and individual differences that may contribute to disagreement and difficulties among caregiving adults. Because we are ultimately concerned with the subjective experience of all participants, the effect of culture on perception and on the meaning of communication styles, childrearing practices, and developmental expectations is intertwined with every aspect of the consultant's work.

Training in mental health consultation is essential for both veteran therapists and newcomers from different disciplines. At Daycare Consultants, the training for new staff is identical to that of graduate student interns. Experience in parent–child treatment and a strong theoretical foundation in development make the transition to a new arena easier. Nonetheless, new application requires new knowledge. Our training incorporates mental health principles and understanding of early childhood education and development.

Most consultants have experience in one of these areas, usually mental health. Training attempts to heighten the trainees' understanding of typical early childhood development and to augment their understanding of group care and its implications for the children's developing sense of self. Enhanced by knowledge of adult group work and organizational functioning, clinical interventions must be adapted to serve as consultative interventions.

Daycare Consultant's training consists of four parts: (a) a didactic training seminar, (b) a clinical conference, (c) clinical supervision, and (d) direct consultation experience.

Didactic seminar

The didactic seminar begins with a focus on observation. Accompanied by a seasoned consultant, trainees observe a variety of child-care settings. We want trainees to begin to appreciate the range of philosophies, environments, and perspectives on child care that exist in the field. We ask them to consider the meaning of their presence on the staff and the ways of initiating the consultation relationship. Training then focuses on recognizing, empathizing with, and responding nonjudgmentally to teachers' particular concerns and their subjective experience. The didactic training seminar also focuses on child development as a transactional phenomenon: A child's sense of self is created and development is influenced by, through, and in relationship.

Clinical case conferences

All consultants-in-training participate in clinical conferences, where they take turns presenting an aspect of their consultative work. Clinical conferences provide opportunities for consultants to discuss shared issues and to receive feedback. Many participants consider the clinical conference one of the most useful aspects of the training. The senior staff and supervisors help facilitate the discussion among the consultants-in-training and generalize from the specific situation being presented to circumstances that impact all the consultants. The clinical conference also offers an opportunity to exchange clinical perceptions; share information regarding resources (community organizations, status of school district programs, possible referrals, etc.); learn about the other consultants' experiences; and commiserate about frustrations, struggles, and disappointments. The clinical conference diminishes feelings of isolation that result from being based in child-care centers or family child-care homes rather than in shared office space as is the norm for most mental health trainees.

Clinical supervision

Individual clinical supervision, in which each consultant-in-training participates for 2 to 4 hours every week, embodies some of the most important aspects of the consultants' training. It provides a place for the consultant to learn about her role and to reflect, focus on, and understand her particular impact in relation to specific centers, families, clients, and situations. A consultant's distress, helplessness, or sense of responsibility may mimic that of the consultees. Supervision offers a space to listen for and attend to these reverberating realities. Clinical supervision helps consultants maintain emotional equilibrium as the supervisor understands and empathizes with the supervisee's conflicting emotions and perspective, just as the supervisee must do with child-care staff, families, and children. The supervisor also fosters mutual exploration and problem solving in the hope that these values are passed from consultant to child-care teacher. This mutual exchange supports high-quality attention to teachers, children, and families. Supervisors focus on three key relationships: the supervisor and the supervisee, the supervisee (consultant) and the consultee (teacher), and the teacher and children for whom she cares. The parallels between each relationship and the others are identified and explored in supervision.

Beginning consultants meet with more than one clinical supervisor. Although all of the supervisors are versed in, experienced in, and share the same fundamental theoretical approach, each brings his or her unique way of seeing and being to the work. This range of perspectives not only affords consultants-in-training experience with various opinions and styles but also supports them as they learn to appreciate infinite variety and develop their own consultative persona.

This Book

Mental health consultation to child care is about, and happens through, relationships. Thus every consultation will be different. Diversity among consultees as well as individual differences among consultants contribute to variations in the consultation experience. We have learned, however, that some basic tenets and practices underlie our consultative efforts. This book attempts to outline our approach philosophically as well as practically.

The central tenet of mental health consultation to child care is what we call the "consultative stance." (Others might call consultative stance a "way of being" or "how you are.") The consultant's stance—her way of being—is founded upon a deeply held belief that the ways in which people are treated influence their views of themselves and, in turn, their relationships with others. Thus Jeree Pawl advises, "Do unto others as you would have others do unto others (Pawl & St. John, 1998, p. 7)." How the consultant is—her demonstrations of interest, empathy, respect, and understanding—is central to successful consultation. Respect and empathy in the consultant's relationships with caregivers positively influence caregiver–child relationships. Caregivers will accept and use the consultant's knowledge in direct proportion to the level of trust and mutual respect established between them. In chapter 1, we describe in more detail the consultative stance that threads through all of our consultative efforts. We also describe the range of activities that is part of mental health consultation in child care.

The remainder of the book is divided into two parts. The first section (chapters 2–5) examines program consultation and how one establishes the consultation relationship and considers the meaning of behavior in that mode of consultation. Several relationships that characterize program consultation are examined: the consultant's relationships with the child-care program's director and staff, the relationships among staff members, and the staff's relationships with parents.

The second section of the book (chapters 6–9) examines case consultation closely. We explore the integration of information from observation and from the adults in the child's life as a way to understand the meaning of a child's behavior. We also examine the process of translating this understanding into responsive action, thereby ameliorating a child's distress.

We hope that this introduction has made our guiding principle clear: Relationships are important. Mental health consultants in child care work toward improving caregivers' self-efficacy, adult–child relationships, and, ultimately, the quality of each child's experience in child care. It is through the consultation relationship that these goals can be accomplished.

Throughout this book, we offer discrete examples of practice to illustrate particular points. In addition, to convey the length and complexity of the consultation relationship, we have created two fictional child-care programs, each an amalgamation of our mental health consultation experiences. In the first chapters, the fictional consultant faces the challenges of program consultation at Bread and Jam Child Care. A single child's experience at the Good Days Child Care Center illustrates case consultation. In each of these stories, we look closely at the consultant's interactions and suggest possible meanings for behavior of the children and the adults.

Although we know that no single endeavor anticipates all the permutations of the consultation relationship, we hope that this book makes navigating the terrain possible and more pleasurable.

References

Knitzer, J. (1996). Meeting the mental health needs of young children and their families. In B. A. Stroul (Ed.), *Children's mental health: Creating systems of care in a changing society* (pp. 553–572). Baltimore: Paul H. Brookes.

Pawl, J. H., & St. John, M. (1998). *How you are is as important as what you do . . . in making a positive difference for infants, toddlers and their families.* Washington, DC: ZERO TO THREE: National Center for Infants, Toddlers and Families.

Yoshikawa, H., & Knitzer, J. (1997). *Head Start mental health strategies to meet changing needs.* New York: National Center for Children in Poverty Columbia University, Mailman School of Public Health, and the American Orthopsychiatric Association.

Chapter 1

Principles, Practices, and the Consultative Stance

Child care is a complicated undertaking. Children spend hours away from their parents in the constant company of other children and several serially shifting adults. For a growing number of young children, this arrangement begins before they may be ready for extended separation or for the intensity of multiple peer interactions. Child-care providers work alone or extremely closely with others. More than in most professions, child-care providers must collaborate, share space, and coordinate every part of their day—a challenge that is beyond many two-parent families, let alone a group of staff members with varied histories, experiences, cultures, and beliefs about children.

Child care is an industry that must adhere to local, state, and federal guidelines as it attempts to make a profit. Child care is an undervalued and poorly compensated profession, in which workers must deal with low wages, little respect, and the demands of their own lives. The parents who need child care the most or for the longest hours typically live in poverty and under stress. With the increase in the use of child care for children across the economic spectrum, many more children are coming to child care demanding special attention from adults who are already overtaxed. In an attempt to meet the individual and diverse needs of all children, approaches to child care vary, from the most structured academic preschool to the most relaxed child-directed day care. The success or quality of these attempts varies even more wildly from custodial to compassionate care.

Whatever the child-care setting, the quality of the relationships among the adults and children can enrich or detract from a child's experience. Although relationships are important in most professions, relationships in child care directly shape young children's growth and development—for good or ill. As more and more very young children spend longer and longer hours in child care, they develop increasingly more significant relationships with their child-care providers. Mental health consultation, designed to enhance all of the relationships in a child-care community, pays special attention to those between caregivers and children.

Consultative Stance

The consultation relationship has the power to transform the other relationships in the child-care system. This relationship's power, we believe, derives from the consultant's "way of being"—her consultative stance. Although consultation is as unique as the persons or programs providing it, we have identified 10 elements that seem to be essential to the consultative stance.

1. Mutuality of endeavor. Consultation can only be effective when the consultee contributes to and participates in the process. Although child-care providers and parents often want immediate answers in times of distress, consultants convey the necessity of constructing hypotheses together. Consultants observe children for relatively brief periods of time; consequently, a full understanding of a child's experience with his caregivers is possible only with the input and participation of those caregivers. Without the caregiver's contribution in the formulation of the problem, and later the plan or response, the likelihood of the caregiver's participation decreases dramatically. A consultant's advice, no matter how intelligent and how "right," is useless if it does not consider the caregiver's perspective and understanding (influenced by individual history, culture and previous experiences with other children and this child) of the situation and, ultimately, the caregiver's willingness to participate in particular changes.

2. Avoiding the position of expert. If one accepts that our work is a collaborative effort between consultant and providers and parents, the expert stance must be abandoned. This is not to suggest that the consultant does not have crucial knowledge about child development, child care, and mental health; however, a full understanding and resolution of a difficulty can only be achieved through gathering information from all the participants. Convinced that positive change occurs only as a truly collaborative relationship develops, the consultant seeks to legitimize and heighten the child-care providers' sense of their own expertise. The consultant is neither shy to offer her expertise nor to receive it from the consultees, but she integrates these perspectives to make them most useful. The consultant knows that there is always more to know. She has ideas based on what, up to this point, she has learned from the participants. Because her attitude conveys her belief that the providers hold valuable ideas, the child-care staff come to see themselves as the source of ideas. In this context, they become aware of the mutuality of the consultative endeavor developing hypotheses together about their challenges and the skills to tackle future difficulties.

Avoiding the position of expert becomes increasingly difficult during crises in the child-care setting and when consultants are new. Anxiety about children's safety or one's ability to offer adequate assistance forces both caregiver and consultant to extremes that ultimately ignore the complexity of a particular situation. For instance, a provider cries that a "biter" is ruining her program, and she needs immediate results as several parents have threatened to remove their children, who have been victims of the biting, from the child-care program and to notify licensing of the unsafe situation. She fears that the "biter" will cause economic hardship for the program, not to mention the fact that her failure to curtail the biting makes her question her ability as a teacher. She demands results from the consultant, and without them she labels the consultant a failure and useless. Faced with a desperate ultimatum for immediate change, a consultant can be convinced that a bit of expert advice will remedy the problem. Avoiding the pull to proffer our expertise is especially important in such situations, as the offer is doomed to disappoint.

3. Wondering instead of knowing. "Wondering with, not acting upon," (Jeree Pawl, 1997 personal communication) the caregivers with whom we are consulting elicits their involvement in the process and properly preserves the sense of the consultee as the holder of essential information and knowledge and as the agent of change. The consultant's stance of wondering, not knowing, demonstrates to the consultee that understanding is a process, not a moment. What follows then is the importance of wondering aloud with caregivers—slowing down the providers and parents, and sometimes, the consultant, to consider the myriad reasons for a child's behavior. Often the way that behaviors are labeled immediately assumes the cause. For example, a child who hits is labeled aggressive, locating the cause of the behavior solely within the child. The relief felt in locating the problem, especially when it is outside oneself, makes holding the stance of wondering, of not knowing, a particular challenge for the consultant—both in response to the appeal of stressed-out caregivers and to the internal desire to be helpful and to relieve pressure in the caregivers. Understanding the caregiver's subjective experience of the child is essential. When consultants are able to hold this stance the benefits are threefold: (a) the complexities of the situation are understood, and a response can consider the child's needs as well as the adults' needs; (b) the caregiver has the experience of participating in the solution giving her greater confidence in her role and ability to affect change; and (c) the consultant instills the idea that relationships affect children's behavior, that patience in the face of crisis is a response, and, most importantly, that "not knowing" is not incompetence but a momentary experience that precedes understanding.

4. *Understanding another's subjective experience.* The consultant introduces the importance of "not knowing" by demonstrating this behavior in her relationship with the caregiver. When the consultant fully accepts that the caregiver holds expert information about her own and the children's experience, the consultant begins the process of understanding the caregiver's subjective experience. One of the frustrations consultants face are child-care staff who are well trained in early childhood education and are unable at times to include this knowledge in their work with particular children. We have come to understand that training alone does not affect change in caregivers. Our experience in infant mental health helped us anticipate that a caregiver's understanding of a child, as well as herself, is just as crucial to creating change as any expertise we, or they, might possess. Sometimes, this requires exploration of a caregiver's history and experiences of parenting and childhood to uncover obstacles to employing the knowledge a provider possesses. Not only does this appreciation for the caregiver's subjective experience create an alliance, it often elicits understanding of attitudes, beliefs and practices that are negatively influencing the caregiver's interactions with children. These obstacles are addressed in consultation.

5. *Considering all levels of influence.* In addition to the personal histories of child-care providers, there are numerous other influences on their view of a child and their ability to assist a child. Although some are internal (intrapsychic), many of these influences are external, including programmatic and bureaucratic pressures and program philosophies. Additional influences are interpersonal. At the interpersonal level, each provider's relationship with her coworkers, administrators, the parents, and the other children affect the possibilities for a relationship with a specific child. The provider–child relationship cannot be meaningfully considered or addressed separately from the many systems within which it exists. The consultant must strive to consider and to understand all these levels of influence affecting the child-care providers' perceptions of children.

6. *"Hearing and representing all voices"—especially the child's* (Pawl, 2000, p.5). Eliciting the voices of all child-care community members, the consultant is dedicated to hearing about and from each individual. Whenever necessary, the consultant represents the perspective of one participant to another with the eventual aim of increasing the adult's capacity to and belief in the usefulness of communicating directly to one another. The consultant promotes the possibility by demonstrating that various views can be held and heard equally. Her goal is not to negotiate a particular outcome but to enlist cooperation, based on understanding, among those involved in children's lives.

Most important, the consultant gives voice to those who literally have no words—the children. While addressing the obstacles, internal or interpersonal, of the adults focusing on the child, the consultant is also assisting to create a holding space in which the children's experience, development, and needs can be meaningfully considered. Consequently, one of the important roles of the consultant is to amplify the voices of children so that their experience can be included and appreciated in solutions and in the daily functioning of a program.

7. The centrality of relationships. Because we know that mental health is promoted through interactions between child and caregivers, the centrality of relationships underlies all of our beliefs about consultation. Understanding caregivers' subjective experiences and giving voice to children's experiences helps us to realize fully the complexities of the relationships and interactions. Child care increases the number of relationships in a child's circle of experience to include more caregivers in addition to parents. For the wheel of development to turn smoothly with the numerous supplemental relationship spokes from the central child, the adult relationships on the circumference must be interlocked.

To illustrate briefly, let us consider an 18-month-old who has difficulties with regulation and who challenges his child-care providers beyond their abilities to comfort him when frustrated, assist him through transitions, and soothe him enough to nap. His parents separated during the pregnancy and have since waged a bitter custody battle that led to an arrangement that requires the toddler to change homes every 3.5 days. Angry with the child for taking an "unfair" amount of their time from other children, the child-care providers report to the parents daily about the problems during the day, unintentionally fueling the acrimony between them. With some understanding and empathy for the staff, the consultant helps to shift the focus to the child's experience. Understanding the obvious contributors to his current functioning allows them to re-energize their empathy for the child. Consequently, they can notice with the parents that the days of home changes are more intense for this child—directing the parent's attention to the shift in homes rather than the "bad parenting" of the other. With this refocusing the parents are better able to communicate with each other first through the staff and later in person with support from the providers and the consultant. Finally, rather than using the child care as the sole transitional space between homes, the parents, with the consultant's assistance, are able to develop a plan that includes both parents more fully creating a consistent experience for their child. In bringing the attention to the child, the consultant with the child-care providers helped the parents redefine their relationship from resented competitors to cooperative partners transforming the 18-month-old's experience as well as their own.

In consultation, we focus on the spokes, and simultaneously attend to the adult relationships forming the ring around the child, as they are crucial to the child's developing sense of self. The strength of those bonds affects the child's experience of continuity. Therefore relationships between parents, between parents and providers, and between multiple providers in a child-care setting become the focus of consultation nearly as often as the relationships between children and their caregivers (parents and child-care staff). Vital to all successful consultation is an appreciation of the ways in which relationships influence other relationships.

8. Parallel process as an organizing principle. The consultants' way of being emanates from her conviction that the ways in which people are treated affect how they will feel about themselves and treat other people. She "do[es] unto others as [she] would have others do unto others" (Pawl & St. John, 1998, p. 7). As the consultant respects, values, and understands the consultee, the caregiver in turn becomes better able to respect, value, and empathize with the experiences of the children for whom she cares. Parallel process extends in all directions and beyond the consultant–consultee relationship. Therefore, the consultant not only behaves as she hopes others might, she encourages such characteristic ways of being among all—directors, parents, and staff.

Most clinicians are trained to identify the parallel processes that occur in the therapist–supervisor relationship as reflections of the client–therapist relationship, but rarely are the vice-versa influences considered. However, as the number of participating and considered relationships increases, it becomes clear that the effects of parallel process move in all directions. In fact, this is a cornerstone of our approach. The relationship created between caregiver and consultant and its quality absolutely create change in the child–caregiver bond in the same way that a child's behavior in the child–caregiver relationship is strongly influenced by prior relationship experiences, especially the parent–child.

9. Patience. All consultants, but especially new consultants, would like programs to offer quality care immediately. Also, the seemingly horrible circumstances of individual, and sometimes groups of, children compound the urgency for improvement; however, this does not serve the consultation process well. If we believe—and we do—that current relationship functioning is not only affected by knowledge but also by individual perceptions and beliefs influenced by experiences of childhood, parenthood, and life, we must also understand the challenges in uncovering, understanding, and finally changing those perceptions and related actions. Just as we encourage and attempt to foster patience in caregivers' relationships with children, we must also be patient with the child-care providers and parents. Sometimes this means that, in order to maintain our ongoing relationship with a caregiver and our faith in the consultation process, it is necessary that we focus on the future children in her care, not exclusively the children currently in the program. Again, focusing on the mutative factors of relationships, particularly the consultant–caregiver relationship, may provide hope for the consultant who has fostered in a caregiver (through their relationship) the possibility that an empathic relationship can affect change.

10. *Holding hope.* Child-care providers often lose hope in the face of daily, sometimes hourly, crises with challenging children, the demands of a classroom of children and their parents, varying levels of competence in fellow staff members, and long poorly paid hours. Their work sometimes seems unimportant and unappreciated, and they lose sight of their efficacy in helping children change and grow (just as we forget this in our consultation efforts with caregivers). Therefore, in addition to maintaining their own hope and belief in change in a slowly shifting system, the consultant must also hold hope for the child-care providers and parents because she is the only one that regularly has the luxury of stepping out of the seemingly static system to see the possibilities.

Consultation in Action

In addition to the 10 elements that make up the consultative stance, we have identified two types of consultation—case consultation and program consultation. Case consultation involves activities on behalf of an individual child. Program consultation, broader in scope, addresses any aspect of a child-care program's functioning that affects the quality of care for all children. Although we discuss case and program consultation separately in the rest of the book, in reality, case and program consultation overlap. In the examples of consultation that we weave throughout the chapters, we address the complexity of the consultative endeavor, but even these accounts are simplified. So let us stop here to look at a snapshot of a day in the life of a mental health consultant to child care—the shifting roles and focus and choices made throughout a single consultation visit.

Lucille, the consultant for the last few years, arrives at the child care. With prior input and agreement from parents and staff, she has planned to observe a child who she has been following. After observing, she plans to meet with the director to discuss a simmering interstaff conflict. Then, the consultant will meet with a parent whose serious mental health issues make it difficult to trust and interact with the staff.

Upon entering the classroom, the consultant finds a child sequestered from the activities crying on a chair near the door. She has paper towels wrapped around her finger. When Lucille makes a sympathetic face for the girl to the teacher, the teacher announces that the child was dropped off at school bleeding from a deep cut on her finger; they've bandaged it, called the parents (1 hour ago), and are waiting for them to arrive. Lucille indicates her empathy for the staff who feel saddled with more responsibility by parents who exploit them. Although Lucille doesn't normally interact with children in the classroom, she looks to the teacher for permission and then speaks to the child soothingly. After comforting her, the consultant finds an activity for them to engage in to distract her from the blood and the pain. Sufficiently engrossed in a one-arm activity, the girl stops crying. Lucille reminds herself to check in with the staff to see how they perceived her intervention. They were angry with the girl's parents for dropping her off in this condition. Will they see Lucille's action as assistance or an indictment of their competence?

Lucille has a chance to look up. Oscar, the child she is here to observe, is doing better. He yells, "Stop it, or I'll hit you." The staff reprimands him immediately, but Lucille wishes they saw the improvement. He has never stopped himself before. For a child who is easily overwhelmed by his surroundings, this is true progress. She will attempt to convey his experience when she meets with the staff later in the week. She hopes that she also has the opportunity to share this with Oscar's mother.

The interactions with Oscar escalate—the head teacher has taken a toy away from him because he won't share. While shrieking and crying, Oscar hits the teacher and throws any object in reach. Finally, he is removed kicking and screaming by the teaching assistant. The head teacher begins to cry, but Lucille has a hard time comforting her because she is angry for Oscar. She composes herself and suggests that they have the director cover the classroom while the distressed teacher excuses herself. In the open office, the teacher sobs uncontrollably. She feels like a failure because she is unable to work with Oscar and yet she is returning to graduate school specifically to specialize in early childhood special education. She fears that she needs to reconsider and worries that no one on staff respects her. While Lucille consoles her, the scheduled parent arrives for her appointment.

Lucille leaves the teacher, who continues to cry loudly, and speaks with the parent briefly. Because she can't be responsive to both simultaneously and she sees that the parent is more balanced than usual, the consultant quickly decides to ask the parent to reschedule. (Later with her supervisor, she wonders if this may have been an opportunity for this usually overwhelmed self-absorbed parent to see and tolerate the notion that others also have challenges and her needs may not always come first, a struggle even with her own child. Of course, the consultant's slight will take repairing.)

In the meantime, Lucille helps the teacher to decide to go home. This means that the consultant's meeting with the director can't happen for she will be covering the classroom. Before she goes, however, Lucille helps the director to call Oscar's mother and to describe his behavior and what might have happened. Because Lucille has followed this case and has a close relationship with the director, she has permission to acknowledge the staff's contribution to this interaction. Together they find a way to convey Oscar's experience that is respectful to both him and to the staff. The director also trusts that Lucille understands the director's balancing act—catering to the needs of children while managing staffing and scheduling issues. The director has agreed to the teacher's early dismissal despite the inconvenience because she knows that Lucille makes her suggestions with knowledge of the program and everyone's best interest in mind. This doesn't mean that Lucille won't raise the issue at their next meeting.

The teaching assistant who removed Oscar makes sure to say to Lucille, "The head teacher doesn't know what she's doing. Since she came, this place has been falling apart." Lucille acknowledges the frustration of the earlier interaction and her burden but also wonders if they might talk about it together during staff meeting. The relationship between the head teacher and teaching assistant had been strained for a long time. Their compensation is so disparate. The announcement that she will go to grad school has stirred the frustration because the teaching assistant, who really is more skilled and who has hoped to pursue college, hasn't been able to afford the time or cost of school. It hasn't helped their relationship or for that matter Oscar's experience that the head teacher's insecurities has led her to strictly cling to their hierarchical roles. The head teacher has assumed that she should handle Oscar because she is in charge even though the teaching assistant has been more adept at connecting with and containing him.

A mental health consultant in a child-care setting is a crisis manager, therapist, "couple's counselor," child development expert and organizational consultant all at once. Knowing when and how to take on each of these roles in a shifting environment is a consultant's constant struggle. Throughout, the consultant's "way of being" determines her success in each of her roles more than any expertise. In addition to the 10 elements of the consultative stance, the consultant must keep in mind the following general as well as specific principles of mental health consultation.

General Principles of Consultation

Most basically, consultation is an activity in which the person asking for help, the consultee, is assisted in addressing a work problem (Caplan, 1970). Hinted at in this skeletal definition are two agreed-upon aspects of consultation. A request for help underscores that the relationship is voluntary for the consultee and that the consultant possesses relevant knowledge.

The transactional nature of problems

Various consultation approaches conceptualize the "work problem" as residing in either the consultee (the child-care provider or center) or the consultee's client (a specific child). We have found that the problem rarely resides in one party. In our approach, the problems and the solutions are seen as interactional. Even when a difficulty emanates from a particular child or the child-care system, the daily interactions make the difficulties transactional.

The consultant's effective involvement hinges not on ascribing primary responsibility but in understanding and helping to shift the interaction. The consultant observes, inquires, and tries to address obstacles to change in both the child and in the child-care system. Even when consultation is centered on a particular child who is baffling to the caregivers, the focus is *not* solely on the "client." The consultant simultaneously considers the consultee's experience of and contribution to the child's situation. The consultee's subjective experience of the child, her skills, institutional limitations, and other internal and external strengths or impediments are seen as significant to understanding and ameliorating a child's difficulties in child care.

The consultant's position

Key to our approach is the positioning of the consultant. She stands outside of the system's hierarchy, as free as possible from its constraints. From this vantage point, she can assess and address influences on both the child and the caregiving system and understand the child–provider relationship. Her positioning allows her to be responsive to both the client and the consultee—child and child-care provider.

The collaborative nature of consultation

Collaboration underlies all of our consultation approach. Each participant possesses an expertise. Consultants must genuinely respect the child-care providers' knowledge of specific children and their general knowledge of the child-care system and of early childhood education. The consultant's respect for the providers' knowledge and perspective engenders a reciprocal feeling. Mutual trust and respect between consultant and consultee are integral to the consultant's efficacy.

However, consultation should offer more than the collaborative exchange of expertise. The consultant must also genuinely appreciate the relationships she creates. Her ability to listen and respond respectfully to child-care providers determines their willingness to hear and accept the information she offers.

Consultants must hold a double consciousness about consultees, which can be difficult when the nature of collaboration is collegial. The child-care providers are both colleagues and "clients." The child-care provider is a client—not clinically but as a consultee. The consultant does however apply her clinically informed understanding of human behavior to the adults as well as to the children. The consultant is as interested in understanding all that contributes to the child-care providers' experiences as she is in understanding the experience of the children around whom consultation is focused. Her mental health training helps her to remember that expectations, perceptions, and behaviors are complexly determined by past and present experiences.

These general principles of consultation are employed and expanded upon in our approach. Consultation may focus on a "client" —a specific child—or on a more general program issue with which child-care providers are struggling. The fundamental principles remain the same whether case or program consultation. Attending to and improving the quality of relationships in child care is the organizing principle informing all consultative endeavors.

Specific Principles and Practices of Mental Health Consultation

Understanding the influences on the formation of any relationship is of course complex. The task is exponentially increased when one must consider the myriad influences in child care. Therefore, the consultant seeks to understand as much as possible about the culture of a particular center. Through direct questioning and observation, she learns about a program's guiding philosophy, daily routines, bureaucratic influences, and interstaff and parent–staff relationships. The consultant must develop an understanding of each provider's role expectations, emotional capacities, and beliefs about development, as these are inevitably expressed in the provider's attitude toward and relationship with children. In turn, these situations create feelings in the caregiver. It is in the context of such nesting relationships, unfolding within the reality of schedules, licensing regulations, cultural expectations, and individual propensities and foibles that consultation takes place.

Use of the relationship

The consultant uses her relationship with the child-care provider to address and to discover the connections between all of these interlocking relationships. Therefore, the consultant must be concerned with her impact on the caregivers because this relates in meaningful ways to the providers' impact on the children. The consultant must understand not only the concerns about a particular child or program issue but also the feelings that these situations create in the caregiver. Through the relationship with the consultant, the caregiver comes to feel that her subjective experience is valued and understood, and she in turn becomes better able to value and empathize with the experiences of the children. Ultimately, consultation's primary goal is to increase awareness and understanding of each child's experience.

Long-term consultation

Our approach assumes that the ways in which people are treated affect the ways they will feel about themselves and treat other people. An understanding of mutually influencing interaction is acquired only over time. Therefore we offer open-ended long-term consultation. By meeting regularly, usually weekly and over an extended period of time, the consultant becomes part of the web of relationships which makes up the culture of the center, affording the best opportunity to be useful to all of the children, families, staff, and administrators. When crises arise or a troubled or troubling child presents himself, the consultant can immediately attend to the pressing concern. She knows the context and is trusted by consultees; consequently her help is more readily absorbed. Over time we are able to assist caregivers in identifying and overcoming obstacles to providing quality care by proactively considering the mental health of all children and working in collaboration with one another and parents on behalf of the children in the program.

Case Consultation and Program Consultation

Earlier we presented the story of one mental health consultant's morning at a child-care center in which program and case material were tightly interwoven as they mostly are in actual practice. Program and case consultation often occur simultaneously. Indeed, the overarching principles of consultation apply to both case and program consultation. Particular practices relate to the specific content of each type of consultation.

We describe case consultation first because child-care programs usually request services around an individual child even when program consultation may become the focus.

Case Consultation

Caregivers often seek services for the first time when they are especially worried, alarmed, or frustrated by the behavior of a particular child. This is especially true of caregivers who have not had opportunities to receive consultation and may feel that the usefulness of consultation is limited to these particularly acute situations. Their feelings of desperation provoke them to seek help when they might otherwise not feel the need. Even as the eventual goal of consultation is to improve the overall quality of care for all children, initially the consultant responds to a provider's immediate needs. When a caregiver has questions or concerns about a specific child, case consultation is offered.

When a particular child is the focus of consultation, we involve the child's parents from the beginning. The consultant may initially merely think with the child-care providers about the least threatening and most useful way to introduce the consultation services to the family. However, specific information about the child is shared with the consultant only with the parents' knowledge and consent.

Taking time to involve parents may be perceived by providers as an impediment to the immediate assistance they desire. Barriers to parent involvement include the lack of an established relationship with the parent or parents' resistance to the identification of concern about their child. First, the consultant thinks with providers about their relationship with the family and developing ways to overcome the mutual mistrust or antagonism.

The consultant's attitude toward and inclusion of parents influences the staff's consideration of the overall importance of their relationships with parents. Only as all of the adults involved in the child's life truly trust the others' intentions can they engage in the process of considering the child's experience and needs. Case consultation relies on such cooperation.

Then, with parental consent, the consultant observes the child in the child-care setting establishing frequency and timing with the child-care providers. Responding to the caregiver's wishes and perspective underlines the consultant's respect for the provider's knowledge of the child.

These observations enable the consultant to evaluate the child's abilities, limitations, vulnerabilities, and strengths. A variety of caregiver–child interactions shed light on the goodness of fit between the child's needs and the program. The luxury of being uninvolved in these interactions allows the consultant to identify antecedents to behavior. Unlike the caregivers, the consultant does not face the demands of a group, allowing her to focus on an individual child. Developing a complete picture relies on the consultant's ability to elicit and integrate the long-standing perspective of the providers and parents with these observations. The consultant meets with all of the adults in the child's life.

Who is involved, the course, content, and even the whereabouts of these meetings are determined mutually and based on the particulars of each situation. Our desire to convey to parents that their participation in the consultation is vital to our understanding of their child is also communicated through our intentional flexibility in when and where we offer to meet them. Although we might meet them at the child-care center at pick-up time or at their office during lunch hour, it often is most convenient to meet with them in their homes as it is the place in which families usually feel most comfortable and in charge of the process. Home visits also provide an opportunity to observe the child in another environment. Seeing similarities or differences in how a child feels, interacts, and behaves in various settings often contributes useful data. Inherent in all exchanges is the sense that the parent possesses information that is essential to our understanding of the child. The consultant is communicating that the child's behavior in child care can be meaningfully considered only as we are able to establish its relevance in connection to all other aspects of the child's experience. Throughout this exploratory endeavor with the parents the consultant makes explicit the intent of her inquiry, linking what she is learning to the goal of improving the child's experience in child care.

Sometimes the problems contributing to a child's distress extend beyond the child-care setting. When exploration with parents reveals a need for additional or longer-term help, the consultant suggests possible referrals for services and follows the family through the process to ensure their engagement. For instance, a consultant may shepherd a family through an assessment for entry into an early intervention program. At other times, assistance is provided in visiting prospective kindergartens or therapists to ensure a comfortable transition.

Again, the quality of the consultant's relationship with a parent affects the parent's openness and trust in other relationships. The consultation relationship facilitates confidence in the referral and willingness to pursue outside resources. The positive experience with a mental health professional, who values parents' contribution and reserves judgment, builds faith in and openness to future therapeutic relationships.

Concurrent to the parent meetings, the consultant is meeting with the child-care providers. The information that a caregiver is able to provide about the child, whether confirming of or differing from the parent's perception, is invaluable to understanding the child's experience. Children who are experiencing difficulties and consequently are difficult to care for arouse feelings of anxiety, anger, and self-blame. As the caregiver begins to feel that the consultant understands and empathizes with these feelings and does not judge, her empathy for the child increases. Concomitantly, trust and mutual respect between the consultant and consultee develops.

Within this relationship the consultant's more didactic developmental information and mental health expertise can become useful in expanding the providers' perspective about a particular child's difficulties. The consultant can then help the caregivers interpret and understand the meaning of behaviors that previously puzzled or frustrated them.

Freeing providers to consider the meaning of a child's behavior is a crucial first step. Genuinely appreciating that all behavior has meaning and simultaneously exploring the idiosyncratic meaning of a particular child's behavior is central to our approach. The consultant's observations in tandem with the information she acquires from the child's parents is usefully distilled and added to the caregivers'. Combining these sources of information allows the consultant and staff to develop possible hypotheses about the meaning of and contributing influences on the child's behavior.

As the child's behavior becomes more comprehensible, caregivers are better able to respond empathically and effectively, engendering the belief that their relationships with children can be agents of change. As caregivers recognize the centrality of their relationships with children, they are more able to consider new ways of interacting. The consultant translates the, now, mutually held understanding of the child's needs into responsive action by incorporating her expertise.

How we offer our ideas is as important as what we are suggesting. The consultant inquires about the feasibility and sensibleness of her suggestions to gauge the providers' enthusiasm and willingness in constructing interventions. As the consultant considers the interventions that might assist a child, she assesses the program's ability and potential to enact them. She remains aware of the constraints of group care. The consultant must acknowledge that, no matter how well she feels she knows a particular program, provider, and child, there may be aspects of the situation about which she is unaware that make her suggestions inappropriate or undoable. Inevitably, the success of any intervention is dependent on the caregiver's genuine sense of its usefulness. Even the most brilliant intervention is doomed to fail if the caregivers are not convinced of its merit. Involving providers in creating an intervention strategy for a child affords the greatest possibility of success. The consultant hopes to instill the belief that one's actions toward children are effective and crucial.

Program Consultation

Establishing a relationship with caregivers, relieving their anxiety and self-doubt, helping them to explore the expectations that influence their relationships with children, and providing didactic information at the appropriate time can improve the care that providers are able to offer to all children. It is often true that in the course of a consultation around an individual child, caregivers themselves recognize this connection. Although they may initially request consultation around one particularly troubled child, they discover that the usefulness of understanding a child's feelings and needs are not limited to a particular case. This realization and the benefits derived from the consultation process often lead to requests for program consultation.

In program consultation the scope of discussion broadens beyond the individual child. Our experience has demonstrated that the factors influencing quality of care and therefore addressed in program consultation are myriad and far-reaching. As the quality of care is, in our view, integrally linked to the quality of relationships within a child-care community, we seek to consider and address all that influences these relationships. Meeting individually and then securing therapy for a provider whose experience with a child in her care has resurrected memories of her own childhood abuse or sorting through a scheduling snafu that has contributed to a staff insurrection are within the realm of issues addressed in program consultation.

Addressing the various levels of a program's functioning

Although the range of activities is wide, the consultant is anchored in her commitment to address all levels and aspects of a program's functioning that influence the quality of care. This may mean involvement at the bureaucratic, interpersonal, or intrapsychic level. She proceeds from the premise that the experiences, past and present, of each individual within the child-care community as well as the systems in which they are currently working relate to the quality of the provider–child relationship: how children are seen, experienced, and cared for.

Setting the parameters of the relationship

A consistent and often longstanding involvement with a child-care program evolves incrementally. This begins by determining with the staff when and with whom we will meet. Establishing a forum for dialogue is a necessary but often arduous first step. The majority of child-care programs with whom we consult did not initially have staff meetings. Having little opportunity to think together about children or program issues is in and of itself a contributing factor to interstaff and programmatic difficulties. Often, minor misunderstandings have escalated into the providers' entrenched mistrust of one another. Through regular meetings with the staff, the consultant assists in untangling the knots of misperception. Establishing meetings and helping staff to see the usefulness of them may then be an important initial goal of program consultation. Understanding all of the intricacies of a child-care community as they impact program functioning occurs only over time. Therefore, the consultant meets with staff regularly for as long as they find our involvement useful, usually years.

The range of focus

The consultant attempts to respond to all aspects of a program that impact quality, but she ultimately aims at enhancing the provider–child relationship. She may address adult interactions, organizational functioning, individual agonies, or the more practical program practices. She may be asked to amend a naptime routine in which no one rests or to think through aspects of the environment that contribute to congestion and chaos. She may help staff understand and implement developmentally appropriate program practices. Whether with an individual or large group, in constructing space for play or a place for a provider's perspective to be voiced, the consultant is committed to understanding and addressing the myriad relationships influencing caregivers as she imagines this will directly relate to the quality of their relationships with children.

Focus on adult relationships

Consultation around adult relationships, specifically those influencing organizational functioning (e.g., interstaff relationships, communication of role expectations, etc.), is a primary focus of our program consultation. Those programs reporting the greatest degree of organizational difficulty prior to consultation were also rated as having the lowest overall quality of care (Pawl & Johnston, 1991). The consultant is assisting individuals within a child-care community to acknowledge their subjective experience and its impact on their work. In so doing, she fosters providers' appreciation of the subjective experiences of her coworkers. Within the established forum, the consultant seeks to assist staff in being able to convey and to hear each other's perspective. As caregivers feel understood and able to understand each other, the quality of their relationships generally improves. In turn, their relationships with children are likely to improve.

Summary

Both case and program consultation rely on and seek to impact adult–child relationships. Which relationships and the content considered differs, but the principles underlying both consultative efforts are the same. The consultative stance threads through both and assists in establishing relationships with providers that serve to improve their existing relationships with each other and the children and their parents toward improvements in the quality of care for all children in a child-care program.

In this chapter, we outlined components of the stance integral to all aspects of consultation: remembering the mutuality of the endeavor, contributing expertise without presuming to be the expert, wondering not knowing, understanding another's subjective experience, considering all levels of influence, hearing and representing all voices, holding the centrality of relationships, holding parallel process as an organizing principle, remaining patient, and holding hope. These are important to the consultant–consultee relationship and by association all other relationships in the focus of consultation. Underlying all of our consultation efforts is the knowledge that the ways in which people are and have been treated affect the ways that they treat others.

References

Caplan, G. (1970). *The theory and practice of mental health consultation.* New York: Basic Books.

Pawl, J. (2000). The interpersonal center of the work that we do. In *Responding to infants and parents: Inclusive interaction in assessment, consultation, and treatment in infant/family practice* (pp. 5–7). Washington, DC: ZERO TO THREE: National Center for Infants, Toddlers, and Families.

Pawl, J. H., & Johnston, K. (1991, August 12). *Daycare Consultants Program final report to the Stuart Foundation: Process evaluation report.* San Francisco.

Pawl, J. H., & St. John, M. (1998). *How you are is as important as what you do . . . in making a positive difference for infants, toddlers and their families.* Washington, DC: ZERO TO THREE: National Center for Infants, Toddlers, and Families.

Chapter 2

Initiating Consultation

After considering the overarching principles of our consultation approach, it is tempting to jump right into the heart of consultation. Throughout consultation, however, we stop action to wonder about what our words and deeds might mean to all participants. We consider—and apply—the principles of mental health consultation before we ever enter the child-care environment. Consultation begins with the request for services. Although it is impossible to anticipate accurately all of a particular child-care program's expectations of consultation, the consultant will bring the tone of "wondering" that will characterize her work with child-care providers to the first intake interview.

In this chapter, we explore the process of beginning consultation in a child-care center. We describe consultants as they enter child-care programs that have never received mental health consultation before and new consultants who are beginning work at centers that have received consultation in the past. Starting with the initial contact and describing a thorough intake process, we offer a series of questions for the consultant that will help to set the appropriate tone and establish expectations.

Among other issues in the initial stages, we will anticipate how child-care staff might (a) interpret the consultant's appearance on the scene (by invitation or intrusion by an administrator); (b) assume the consultant's purpose (to help, criticize, evaluate, report) and position (expert, outsider, supporter); and (c) guess the consultant's charge ("fix" a kid, settle staff disputes, etc.). Considering all of the possibilities helps direct a consultant's entry into a child-care program.

Initial Request

The way in which we enter a child-care program will have lasting effects on a program's receptivity to and understanding of consultation. Directors and staff make immediate judgments about the consultant's usefulness that affect their on-going perceptions of the work and the relationship. When discussing children, we attempt to convey to child-care providers that all behavior has meaning. We hold ourselves to the same standard in our consultative efforts—a consultant's behavior will have meaning to child-care providers just as their behavior conveys meaning. Together the behaviors and perceptions of each create a working relationship.

Careful attention to these details from the very beginning of consultation increases our understanding of each other and the effectiveness of consultation. We reserve judgment until we have had an opportunity to understand the circumstances that contribute to the providers' behavior—among them, current conditions in the center, life history, relationships with coworkers, and beliefs about children.

Through our actions as consultants, directly and indirectly communicated through behavior and words, we hope to achieve a number of outcomes. In the initial contact, we should make sure that several of the essential elements of consultation are present:

1. Our approach of "wondering, not knowing."

2. A sense of understanding and empathy for the adults.

3. Parallel process an organizing principle—the belief that the way that we treat and attempt to understand the adults in a child-care setting will affect their treatment of the children in their care.

Initial Considerations

From the first contact onward, one must pay attention to expectations—the consultant's as well as the program's. From the first phone call, one is negotiating between a program's wishes about our role and our willingness and ability, as consultants, to respond. Particularly when people are in crisis (which often precipitates the request for consultation), the consultee hopes that the consultant will be able to fix their problems. People in crisis are seldom patient. The consultant must balance opposing forces—the wish to be immediately responsive to an expressed need and the desire to understand as much as possible about the situation before proceeding. Considering eight questions can help the consultant begin her work wisely.

1. Can they tolerate the wish to slow down and consider? By the time a child-care program is seeking outside assistance to understand their difficulties, problems seem both insurmountable and intolerable. Stopping to think about how the caller and the program have come to understand the problem and how they will perceive or be prepared for the consultant's entrance will appear to be a waste of valuable time. It is here, however, that one can take the first steps in demonstrating that understanding is a process. "Wondering, not knowing" seems luxurious in the face of overpowering demands, yet it is crucial for full understanding and—ultimately—greater effectiveness. One begins by asking details about the referral itself, while being attentive to the anxiety that questioning creates.

The consultant must balance the provider's and child's needs with the wish to gather useful data. The consultant remains aware of the associated costs of any decision or action. Sometimes, a request for consultation becomes so pressured that one may choose to forego a fuller understanding to relieve anxiety. For instance, the child-care provider may desperately want the consultant to observe a child who is challenging the staff. Understanding the reason would be useful and observing without discussion may have its own costs, but the consultant may decide that the provider cannot initially tolerate the lack of response. The consultant might observe in order to respond to the provider's need that may include, among others, the wish for the consultant to understand their position and the desire to have confirmation of the difficulty. Regardless, the consultant may respond immediately and seek understanding later.

What becomes important is the consultant's awareness of the caller's experience during this intake process. How does the caller tolerate questions? Are the responses thoughtful and engaged or are they frustrated and impatient? Successful consultation requires tracking back and forth between process and content. The caller's reaction to the process determines the consultant's response.

2. What are they asking for? When asking for assistance, a child-care provider usually has some idea (consciously or unconsciously) of how that help should manifest. Their ideas begin to inform us about what they expect of consultation and how they understand and approach problems. For instance, a request to observe a child and meet with parents before meeting with the staff, suggests that the program feels overwhelmed, may not be able to imagine their own efficacy, may not have created an ongoing relationship with parents, and may fear conflict with parents. Such a request also alerts us to their expectation that the consultant has an expert eye and that her observations will be a catalyst for change in the child. Successful intake uncovers the complexity and combination of these reasons.

Although a consultant's ideas of how to begin may deviate from what is requested, awareness of how the interaction unfolds is most important. To continue the above example, the consultant may suggest meeting with the director and staff before observing a child. Although the child-care provider may agree to the arrangement, her initial wish has been denied. In order to acknowledge this possible disappointment—an important demonstration of respect—the consultant must be alert. The consultant tries to remain abreast of the child-care providers' wishes, responds when possible, and acknowledges the provider's frustrations with and feelings about the consultant throughout.

3. Who is inviting you? Most child-care programs have several staff members, only one of whom actually makes the request for consultation. The director (or a particular staff member) wants the consultant's involvement, yet others in the system may not be aware of the invitation or the value of asking an outsider for assistance. Therefore, during the intake, one asks about the staff's awareness of and openness to a consultant. The particular participants requesting services predict the receptivity of the staff as well as the purpose of the request. A request from a director who has not spoken with her staff about the possibility of a consultation intervention may suggest that a program has a well-defined hierarchy. Staff in such a program may assume that the consultant's role is to evaluate their performance. Alternatively, a staff member who calls without the knowledge of the director communicates something different. Among other possibilities such a request may indicate a lack of faith in or respect for the director. If the consultant responds to either of these hypothetical requests without contemplating the effects on everyone in the program, she may jeopardize the success of the consultation by generating serious misunderstandings and failing to fully engage all program participants in the consultation process.

Not everyone imagines that consultation will be useful. Our faith in the process may cause us to forget that not everyone believes that consultation from an outsider, especially a mental health professional, can be useful. The words "mental health" can compound participants' suspicions. To find out about participants' reservations about consultation, the consultant encourages them to express their concerns. A willingness to accept the most ardent resistance demonstrates the consultant's ability to tolerate disagreements and her wish to fully understand the child-care providers. Discovering these worries early and addressing them in initial meetings helps to alleviate some of the providers' fears. Unchecked, the apprehension would challenge the consultant's ability to assist.

In addition, other center staff will have a reaction to the person who has requested the consultant. Understanding some of these relationships prior to first meetings may help to make sense of the dialogue among staff members. Focusing consultative efforts becomes easier for the consultant when she has identified those most open to her contribution and those she has to win over.

Understanding who is making the consultation request directs the consultant to some initial hypothesis about how the consultant's presence will be received and perceived. For instance, a director who feels overwhelmed by her supervising duties and the lack of trained staff may independently seek help, wanting an ally to help oversee and educate staff. Accepting such a role might place the consultant in a potentially contentious relationship with the staff.

4. *Who do they expect you to be?* Before the consultant arrives, staff will have made some assumptions about her, based on her title, her level of education, her agency, and their prior experiences. Even child-care providers who are open to the consultant's appearance in the child-care milieu have varied ideas about how the consultant will be useful. Some will expect the consultant to take over with children and families who are posing challenges. Others will want someone to confirm their choice to expel a child. A few will assume that the consultant has all the answers and will immediately relieve them with targeted information that solves all their problems. Others may just want someone to focus on a particular area—environment, curriculum, or parent trainings—because they have already labeled the problem and have constructed their idea of the most effective response. By identifying staff expectations in the early stages of the consulting process, the consultant can clarify her role and her limitations, minimizing disappointments and misunderstandings.

Occasionally, a program is suspicious of outsiders and does not expect the consultant's presence to be supportive. In these instances, the consultant's entrance is associated with evaluation and added burden. This misinterpretation creates its own challenges and may be a barrier to initial acceptance.

5. *Who holds unrealistic expectations and why?* During the intake or initial phone call, the consultant does not have the opportunity to speak with everyone in the program. The director or other caller, however, can begin to give the consultant clues about individuals and their potential responses to the idea of consultation. A consultant is immediately curious about: Who was involved in requesting support? Who is likely to immediately embrace consultation? How does the caller imagine staff will react to a new person? Have others asked for help?

Discussing the participants and their willingness to join the process helps the consultant anchor herself before docking. More importantly perhaps, the consultant begins to convey the importance of understanding each member of the group—assuring child-care providers that they will be respected and included in finding solutions to problems. Mental health consultation is based on the idea that difficulties, and their solutions, are usually broader than originally conceived. Ideally, everyone in the program participates in gaining an understanding of problems and in devising and testing solutions. By establishing a respectful, inclusive approach in early interactions, consultants prepare child-care providers for the slowing down necessary to greater understanding.

6. *Is there a history of consultation (mental health or otherwise)?* Although every group will have some expectations of a new outside consultant, individuals who have had some experience with consultation will have more clearly defined visions. Their prior experience with outside assistance will directly affect the impending relationship with a new consultant. Did they find the previous consultation useful? How did the relationship with the consultant end, and why?

Staff reactions to a shift in consultants can include, among others, loss or mourning, anger, relief, and anxiety. Comparisons between the new and old consultants are inevitable, and responses are likely to be varied. If prior consultation has been helpful, most child-care directors and staff may greet the new consultant with anticipation and friendliness. However, others might be struggling with the loss of a "member of their team" and resist a replacement. If, on the other hand, past consultation experiences have felt unhelpful, threatening, or even burdensome, a new consultant might face opposition to her arrival.

A new consultant can never fully anticipate a program's response to her arrival. Timing, the current functioning of the program, and the individual psychologies of all participating members interact to shape the overall response. However, understanding as much as possible about a child-care program's past consultation experiences can help a consultant understand the new process as it unfolds, smoothing the inevitable bumps. (These ideas will be revisited in chapter 3.)

7. How do staff perceive the problem that precipitated the request for consultation? As she listens to a caller describe the concerns that have led to the request for consultation, the consultant gains a valuable beginning understanding of how the program approaches problems and how staff understand their roles and relationships with children. When she asks questions about how concerns are viewed, she shows respect for the child-care provider's knowledge. Asking also demonstrates the consultant's view that understanding the myriad contributors to any conundrum precedes a solution. The provider's response reveals something about her understanding of the child or program issue, her level of stress, and her willingness to consider alternative explanations.

Her responses to the consultant's questions shed light on how and where the provider focuses attention. For example, she may describe an aggressive child as a child who was not disciplined enough and has been "spoiled," as a child who may have been abused, or as a child who is "just a bully." A provider's thinking will indicate her feelings about the child and his or her parents, how they have responded to the problem so far, and their ability to empathize with the needs of the child.

As the consultant begins to "wonder" about the various parts of the referring situation, she conveys confidence in the provider's perceptions and knowledge. She also conveys her wish to understand and empathize with the child-care provider's full experience. Finally, she models an inclusive approach to the exploration of concerns from the beginning of the relationship.

8. Who are we? Finally, the services that we have to offer are described. However, the intake consultant has no illusion that telling will translate to immediate comprehension. Consultation is understood only as it is experienced. Questions up to this point have already indicated the consultative approach. In crisis, the caller may not be able to take in the more abstract ideas about relationship and the unfolding process of understanding. Therefore, a concrete description of the activities involved is necessary. This might include observing children and classrooms, helping providers to talk with parents about the wish for a consultant's involvement, or offering a meeting with program staff. A general statement about the goal of these activities is also offered. The intake consultant suggests that the aim is to engage all of the involved adults in better understanding contributors to the current difficulty and together coming up with solutions that suit their setting. Even within this description, we are underlining the importance of their contribution and knowledge in creating solutions.

Referral Types

Each of the questions posed above informs our consultation efforts and attempts to create mutual exchange and understanding toward a transforming consultation relationship. As in all relationships, various circumstances impede or enhance ideal interaction. Let us begin, then, with how the initial request comes. We cannot anticipate all variations, but there are three commonly occurring forms: (a) a request from a director or staff member; (b) a transfer from a previous consultant; and (c) contractual obligations leading to consultation. We will look at how these circumstances affect the process and begin to demonstrate how previous suggestions can be utilized for effective consultation.

Director or staff request

The easiest entrance for a consultant begins with a self-referral from a director or staff member. Even with an invitation, there is plenty of work to do in the early stages to clarify the limits of this invitation. Acknowledged need creates a door for the consultant to enter. Although eventually the problem may be more complex and the resistance of director and staff may be great, the consultant can refer to the original request to root herself in the program.

At this point, asking about how the program has responded to the situation for which they are requesting consultation is important. One receives a history of the difficulties and begins to understand a program's functioning and responsiveness. Because the questioning wonders about their understanding of the source of the dilemma as well as their response to the problem, it also begins to suggest that the challenges are based in relational experiences. This is usually a shift from the perceptions leading to the call. Often, a director calls with a seemingly intractable predicament requiring an immediate response that is usually around a specific child or particular program issue. Rarely is the child-care program identified as an involved participant. For instance, the director wishes to fix the child or family but does not consider that some programmatic challenges may contribute to the child's difficulties.

In addition, we are concerned about who is aware of and involved in the circumstance for which consultation is requested. How much do the parents or for that matter other staff know about their concerns and our possible involvement? Broadening the scope of those involved or considered demonstrates our belief in the transactional nature of problems and solutions but also shows how we plan to treat the participants (or consultees) and demonstrates our expectation for the relationships of the adults in child care.

By the time someone is calling for outside help, the situation often feels critical. The actual seriousness of the crisis may vary depending on the caller, but the perceived seriousness is often the same—something has to be done now. Usually, a caller wants the consultant to observe a child and tell staff what is wrong and how to fix it. Rarely is this the most beneficial beginning, but the wish for instant relief needs to be acknowledged. While empathizing with the need for solutions, we explain the importance of meeting with and understanding the staff (and parents) and their concerns before making any moves to solve the trouble.

The hopes about what the consultant can accomplish are highest when the needs are great; consequently, clarifying the extent of the consultant's involvement is extremely important. Anticipating child-care providers' hopes and eventual disappointments help to stabilize and sustain the relationship. To describe consultation and address these expectations, one might say, "I can appreciate your urgency, it sounds like a daily struggle to survive with this child who needs so much adult support. The last thing you want to hear from me is that consultation cannot work without you, the other child-care providers, and this child's parents' involvement. But I would be remiss and would ultimately disappoint you if we don't come to a mutual understanding of what consultation is and is not. I usually begin the process by getting a sense of the child through conversations with his parents and all of his caregivers. What I learn from these conversations gives me an idea about what to watch for when observing. Then we will put our heads together and see if we can come up with interventions to assist this child."

As always, the tone of consultation is set early. At every turn reasons are being explored. What do the consultees think contributes to their challenges? What have they done to date? How did they make those choices? What has been successful so far? What do they think it will take to fix the problem? From the first interaction, this type of inquiry demonstrates the consultation process.

> Suzie, the director of a small child-care center, calls her local mental health consulting agency. She begins urgently, "I heard that you could send someone out to help us. We need someone immediately."
>
> "What kind of help were you looking for?" asked the intake coordinator.
>
> Suzie described how she had to protect her staff from 3-year-old Natasha. "That sounds very upsetting. Protect your staff?" asked the coordinator. Suzie began to describe how Natasha had bitten and hit staff and children. Her mother blamed it on the staff, but they knew that she had been excluded from two other child-care settings in the last year. Worrying about the child, the coordinator says, "Wow, that's a lot of changes for Natasha." The director misses the attempt at empathy for Natasha, "Well, it proves that she needs more help than we can give her." "It does sound overwhelming," says the coordinator shifting her empathy, "How did you hope that we could help?" Suzie hadn't ever worked with a consultant, but had heard from a provider at another child-care center that Daycare Consultants had helped "straighten out" a similarly difficulty situation. When the intake coordinator asked her how her colleague had described the consultant's assistance Suzie admitted she was unsure.

The coordinator briefly explained the general course and components of a case consultation. She talked about observation as well as conversations with providers and parents. She then inquired, "Do you think Natasha's mother would be open to services?" Suzie answered, "Probably not, but I haven't talked to her." "How do you usually have meetings with parents?" The coordinators innocent question was experienced as an accusation. Suzie defensively retorted that the teachers talk to parents at the end of the day, "We'd be meeting everyday if we wanted to tell Natasha's mom about all the problems. We don't have time for that." The coordinator wondered about the staffing and how the afternoon staff finds out Natasha's morning routine. Suzie counters that the problems usually occur during naptime and afterward so that the afternoon staff is there. The intake coordinator focuses on the adult's experience, "That's a hard time in many child-care programs, the staff needs a break and if a child has a hard time with changes or saying good-bye it can disrupt an entire center." "Exactly," exclaimed Suzie.

The intake coordinator offers, "You said that you're not sure how much longer your program can keep Natasha if her behavior continues. Figuring out what Natasha's behavior is telling us and finding ways to help her could take some time and a lot of the staff's energy. Do you think everyone has enough reserve to keep trying? Would you and your staff be able to meet with a consultant? That would give the consultant the opportunity to get the fullest picture possible because the teachers are the experts on the experience with this child. The consultant could join your staff meeting."

Suzie laughed, "I wish we had staff meetings." Staff meetings had not been instituted, and Suzie thought it was hard to imagine having one that included an entire classroom. Only one aide overlapped the two shifts, and the separate staff shifts were having a territorial dispute. Suzie had been afraid to mix the two. Doing so on Natasha's behalf seemed especially daunting as the afternoon staff was ready to say good-bye to her and felt the morning staff blamed them for Natasha's behavior as her difficulties rarely surfaced during their watch.

The coordinator suggested that Suzie meet with the consultant to map out the best strategy for introducing consultation to the staff. Suzie had called because she had wanted to be helpful, but she had requested the services without anyone else's knowledge or input. She was neither sure about the staff's receptivity nor the parent's willingness to participate. They agreed to plan their next move with the tentative hope that Natasha's challenges would be addressed.

The intake coordinator briefed the new consultant. Natasha would serve as the focus, but there were obvious difficulties in the staff relationships. The coordinator and the consultant discussed several possibilities: (a) Suzie may be challenged by supervising and asserting her authority; (b) the staff has personality clashes that impede communication; (c) the morning and afternoon programs function differently, and Natasha responds to those differences; (d) there is a lack of parent inclusion; and (e) although Natasha's emotional difficulties seem to be affected by her school life, there may be some temperamental differences and home experiences that also contribute to her challenges.

The above example illustrates a few important points. When a consultee's only experience with mental health services has been individual services for those in crisis, difficulties will be framed by individual mental health issues. Systemic problems are rarely seen from the inside. Even when told that consultation can address adult needs, rarely do adults choose, at least initially, to focus on themselves. The wish to externalize is universal as is the avoidance of the emotional distress of fully realizing a child's experience (sometimes quite painful) or of one's own contribution to that distress. However, often the adults' struggles are revealed through thorough but empathic questioning.

Although the director was aware of some of the challenges in her program—she laughs at the lack of staff meetings and becomes defensive when questioned about parent contact—she focuses her consultation request solely on Natasha. Natasha's difficulties may have originated with home experiences, but her challenges are likely exacerbated rather than helped in the child care. If Natasha's difficulties are related to transitions, the staff may inadvertently compound the problem by not communicating. Unable to rely on each other, they are unlikely to be able to provide the assistance necessary for Natasha.

The lack of institutional support for staff communication—no staff meetings, little staff overlap between shifts—most likely intensifies the tensions among staff members. This may also create barriers for the consultation and ultimately affects Natasha's functioning. The consultant will have to balance the request for services and the wish to focus on Natasha with efforts to relieve some of the institutional pressures that influence the identified problem.

Suzie also seems to feel powerless to affect change. The coordinator's suggestion that the director meet with the consultant separately hopes to accomplish two goals. The initial meeting with her rather than staff bolsters her leadership position, but the content—considering strategies for staff receptivity and participation—will also help to establish the consultant's stance, specifically the wish to voice the subjective experience of all and to create a collaborative effort. In addition, the consultant will attempt to establish Suzie's support (or lack of) for Natasha's continuing and the decision-making process for excluding a child. This includes how decisions are made, who makes them, and what level of behavior constitutes reasons for expulsion.

It is clear that staff had not participated in the consultation request. As the consultant meets the staff, it will be important to gather the others' wishes for consultation and their interpretation of the problem. The consultant can help Suzie include input from staff in the decision making while respecting her leadership position. Prior consultation was not immediately addressed, but it seems clear that there has been limited if any consultation experience.

Because Suzie has called in crisis about this family, her hopes as well as her staff's may overestimate the consultant's ability to affect change. Clarifying their expectations and creating realistic ones may create initial disappointment but will avoid greater disillusionment and disruptions in the ongoing consultation relationship. Often initial requests for consultation are like this one, at the point of excluding a child. Programs that have not experienced the benefit of consultation call when experiencing an acute crisis. It may not be possible to maintain children like Natasha when problems have become entrenched. In these instances, a secondary goal is necessary—helping the program see that they can seek help earlier in the process, thus averting expulsion for the next challenging child.

Although the coordinator followed the director's lead, she attempted to slow Suzie down to consider Natasha's experience. In these initial moments, she models the stance of wondering—what could contribute to Natasha's behavior? Suzie was not able to tolerate this focus for an extended period, but the coordinator has at least opened up the possibility that behavior has meaning and that the contributors to any behavior are complex but decipherable. Her tone, however, affords a level of respect and compassion for the staff. The coordinator may have different ideas about Natasha and the best way to proceed, but she shows her willingness to consider theirs. By doing so, she has begun the modeling process, hoping to convey the importance of curiosity and compassion for Natasha's tribulations. Even in the initial conversation "levels of influence" are considered and the subjective experience of all participants is noted.

Transfer

Because consultation is often an extended process, there are inevitable shifts in consultants for a child-care program. From time to time, a consultant leaves for other responsibilities—another job, maternity leave, another internship, etc. Transfers affect consultee's feelings about consultation. Planned or unplanned, we hope that the previous consultant was able to anticipate and process the termination. In either case, the new consultant faces challenges. The consultant's inquiries about previous consultation become even more important when she is replacing another consultant. The new consultant needs to convey empathy regarding the loss, the wish for continuity in services, and the desire to know and understand the staff. The latter creates challenges when the staff members have already made themselves known to a consultant. Although they will have some understanding of the consultation process and may make easier use of the consultant's expertise, they may also have difficulty trusting the replacement for fear of losing another supportive person.

In addition, the consultant and the consultees create the consultation process and content together; therefore, consultation with varying consultants will differ even if the intent is the same. There may either be resentment or welcoming of a new consultant depending on previous experiences, which may alternate depending on the staff members in a center. Knowing as much as possible about this before entering and then examining the differences with the consultees solidifies the budding relationships and shows respect for the loss and changes. Again, a parallel to our hope for how the children's experience of transitions are treated is demonstrated right from the start.

If the previous consultation relationship felt beneficial, the replacement benefits from positive institutional transference. However, even when the previous relationship was positive, the new consultant faces particular challenges. Participants often unconsciously assume that the new consultant can take up exactly where the last person left off. Making time for the new consultant to get to know the program, staff, and children is seen as an impediment. She may be perceived as less helpful or knowledgeable than her predecessor. Initially, she is. The entering consultant can avoid these negative attributions by predicting them with the staff. She might try, "After 2 years working with Cynthia, I imagine she knew you and your program pretty well. I hope you'll be patient with my need to ask questions and my desire to spend some time observing in your program. At first, I'm certain that we will move more slowly toward solutions than you were eventually able to with Cynthia, but I'm confident that we can establish a useful consultation connection, too."

Case Example

It may be helpful to look more closely at how consultation actually begins. What follows is a case example based on our experiences. Of course, names and identifying information have been changed to protect our consultees. We have also combined experiences from several programs to shield anyone from being identified. Still, the combination that we present simplifies the complexity of a true consultation for the sake of brevity and understanding. Because we have touted the benefits of long-term consultation, we will follow Bread and Jam Child Care through this and subsequent chapters to illustrate how the consultant's relationship with the providers builds and then provides a foundation that makes interventions easier and more nuanced.

> Bread and Jam Child Care has had two different consultants over the last 2 years. Today, the third consultant, Marsha, calls Patricia, the center director. She seems rushed and annoyed, "I don't have time to meet this week and I'm not really sure if I'll have time next week." Marsha persists, "It must be very busy as the school year begins, I'm sure there are all new kids. I certainly don't want this to be another burden." Patricia retorts, "Well, then we should probably meet after September ends." It was only mid-August and Marsha wondered if the rebuff was related to the last consultant's leaving, "Wow, you're busy. Initiating a new consultant must feel like the last thing you have time for. Had you and the previous consultant established an easy routine?" Patricia responded immediately, "Far from it. I never knew when she was going to come and then she would just expect me to meet with her. I am not even sure what she did." Marsha tried again, "That doesn't seem like it was very useful, and our services should be. Given that experience, I'm thankful you're willing to try again. When you're ready, I would hope to talk about how consultation could serve your center better. It seems like things feel so overwhelming there, and sometimes it's good just to step back and name what you need." Patricia relaxed somewhat, "I suppose you're right." She quickly stiffened before Marsha could begin again. "But I really don't have time," she finished. Marsha thought to herself, "I am

never going to figure out what to do here." Marsha nervously stammered, "Well, in the next 2 weeks, I have a lot of flexibility. I am willing to meet you whenever you think you have a moment." Patricia softened slightly but still tested, "Well, Friday nights are the only openings. Most of the kids are picked up early. I usually begin to close at 5:00 p.m. and go home at 6:00 p.m. If you come at 5:00 p.m., I might be able to see you." Marsha sighed to herself and said, "All right, then I will see you on Friday next week." Patricia sounded surprised, "Okay. I guess I could meet on Friday this week if you're willing." "Absolutely," Marsha happily agreed.

Marsha couldn't wait to get to supervision. She didn't know where to begin, and at least the supervisor knew what the last consultant "really" did. Marsha had been a therapist in a child clinic prior to becoming a consultant. She prided herself on her skills with children who were at-risk socially and emotionally. She seemed to understand the most difficult children and make headway. When her colleagues were challenged, she was the one who provided relief by offering suggestions or sometimes even taking over. Over the years, she had become more and more frustrated, however, as the children who made progress in therapy were returned to the circumstances that contributed to their challenges. She had become better at including parents in the treatment and collaborating with them, but still she had wanted to make a bigger impact. The new Welfare-to-Work regulations had forced most of the mothers of the children that she saw in treatment back to work in subsistence jobs. They were spending fewer and fewer, yet more stressed, hours with their children, and their children were placed in substandard care, exacerbating the family's challenges. The extent of the families' difficulties seemed overwhelming. The idea of making an impact on a child-care center full of children seemed exciting. If she could make the teachers in a few child-care programs understand, a whole bunch of children would have healthy relationships for at least 8 hours a day. She jumped at the chance to become a mental health consultant, but now facing her first challenge, she wondered if she would be able to make a difference.

Sometimes, Marsha was a little impatient. The pace of beginning consultation was not as fast as she would like. She thought her supervisor belabored some aspects of beginning. Supervision was imbued with her wish for rapid change and her frustration when it did not occur. Today, however, she was a little bit relieved things had gone slower than anticipated. Her supervisor could see she was anxious about this first phone call with the center director, Patricia. Marsha explained, "I was as nice and as accommodating as possible, but she just didn't seem to want me to come. I don't know if she will ever want me to be there. What should I do next?"

Her supervisor smiled to herself as Marsha poised her pen ready to write down the "splendid" supervisorial suggestions. Marsha liked answers. She had always done what she was told and was most often very good at it. Like many therapists, she had been and continued to be her family's caretaker, becoming nervous when the next step was unclear. The supervisor realized that they would have to watch for Marsha to lock on answers that relieved immediate anxiety but left the children, staff, or parents inadvertently outside.

"Given what you know so far, what do you think happened?" the supervisor questioned. "For once," Marsha thought, "could she just tell me what she thinks?" She sat quietly for a moment.

"Well," Marsha began, "I know that Patricia is angry." "Angry?" encouraged the supervisor. Marsha momentarily felt some empathy, "I think she feels sort of abandoned. She mentioned more than once that the consultant just left her and was unpredictable. But I can't believe the previous consultant was that irresponsible. We talked before she left, and she seemed conscientious and scheduled appointments way in advance." They considered Patricia's experience—two consultants on whom she relied left abruptly. Even without knowing the director's personal experience of separation, it was clear that the losses would have an impact.

Marsha left her supervisor's office feeling confident and prepared, again remembering that Patricia chose to meet sooner rather than later. Five o'clock on Friday came and Marsha arrived at the center. It was particularly quiet—a few children in their coats outside ready to go. Leticia, the assistant preschool teacher, stood with a few of her charges in tow. Marsha introduced herself and asked for the director. "Patricia left about 20 minutes ago," she said exasperatedly, "leaving me here with this one," pointing to Leo, a 4-year-old. Uncomfortable, Marsha tried to be empathic with Leticia while realizing that Leo could hear every word as he ran around them in circles. She tried, "It's hard to be the only one left to handle tired children at the end of a long day." Leticia foiled her attempts, "It's not the children, it's Leo." Marsha smiled with empathy but did not want to further encourage this conversation. Instead, she introduced herself as the new consultant and shared her wish to be helpful. "Do you have your own children?" asked Leticia. Caught off guard, Marsha answered directly, "No." Leticia revealed proudly that she had nine children. Marsha responded in kind, marveling at her parenting experience and added that Leticia's life experience must have prepared her well for group care. Marsha was tempted to ask more but resisted because she did not want to overstep boundaries while her standing with the director was so precarious, and she so new to the center.

She left a note for Patricia and called on Monday. Patricia had forgotten. They rescheduled for the end of the week—Friday at 5:00 p.m. This time Patricia kept Marsha waiting as she closed some of the classrooms, but they finally met at 5:20 p.m. Marsha felt annoyed but tried not to show it. Patricia, however, didn't have such restraint. Immediately, she began to criticize Marsha's agency for not giving her the services that she had been promised. Marsha squirmed and apologized, but this didn't seem to be satisfying Patricia. Patricia pulled out the contract and pointed to the 5 hours of service they were due and had not been receiving. Marsha resisted the urge to defend and instead expressed empathy for Patricia's perception. Clearly, the previous consultation arrangement was unsatisfactory. She wondered aloud several times what in particular Patricia had hoped would occur in those 5 hours that hadn't, but Patricia repeatedly returned to time not content.

Marsha realized that despite Bread and Jam's 2 years of receiving consultation, the changes in consultants meant that Patricia hadn't really seen the services as beneficial. Marsha assured Patricia that she could spend 5 hours a week, but also suggested that she hoped that together they could figure how best to use this time. Marsha thought perhaps a review of the range of consultation activities she could offer and her particular areas of expertise would help, "Some of the things we could do with the time include discussing children and their parents, interstaff issues, training, and possibly some individual services for children. We could talk about what might be most useful and how you want to apportion my time." For the first time, Patricia seemed to relax. Surprised by Marsha's willingness to cede control, Patricia struggled as she tried to name her preferences.

Marsha rescued her, and Patricia seemed to appreciate having help. "Perhaps we should talk about what worked and what wasn't useful about your previous consultation experience. That might help us to know where to begin." With the new focus, Patricia began to talk about the services with parents that seemed most useful. As Patricia recalled the past, she reminded herself how consultation had been helpful. She had actually liked the last consultant but felt like the ending was abrupt. "Of course," Marsha empathized, "most people have a hard time with good-byes especially when they're unexpected. You've been so busy, you haven't had the time to reflect about it." Patricia quieted, and Marsha flashed on her earlier hypothesis that other experiences of loss could be contributing to the intensity of Patricia's response to the consultant's departure, which may have been perceived as abandonment. The director stiffened quickly, "So, you should spend your 5 hours observing children and picking out the ones who are in trouble. Come early so you can introduce yourself to parents." They had just slowed down and now they were speeding up again. Marsha was torn—if she responded to Patricia, she might alienate staff by intruding on their classroom, but at the same time her relationship with Patricia was so shaky that if she didn't respond she would risk the truce they had just brokered. She was tempted to ask Patricia about the shift in mood but resisted in deference to their tentatively established connection.

"I would be happy to observe, but before we do that I'd like to know exactly what you would like me to see. You and your staff know the children best so maybe you can direct me so that my observations are more focused," tried Marsha.

"I don't know when we could do that. You could just start observing and we'll meet later."

Marsha wondered aloud, "I don't know the staff yet, what do you think they'll make of my arriving unannounced in their classrooms?" Patricia said that most of them would easily accept it, as they always have people dropping in, like licensing, accreditation assessors, and prospective parents. Marsha wondered if what she was hearing boded badly for beginning and said, "Sounds like all of the other folks you mentioned have evaluation as their reason for observing. I suppose the staff couldn't help but see me in the same role. If they saw me as judging their teaching, I worry we'd be off to a less than comfortable start. Just like you and I need to spend some time sorting out who a consultant can be, I would want the staff to get an accurate idea about my role and I would like to know a bit about them. Maybe you could help me to get a sense of the staff before I meet them. If we can't have a meeting, at least I'll know something about them and then maybe you can tell them about me before I go into the classroom."

Patricia began to tell Marsha about the staff, starting with Tyra. Tyra, one of the toddler teachers, was wonderful with the children but seemed to fight with every adult including Patricia. Bob, the other toddler teacher, pushes Tyra's buttons because he is much more laid back. Leticia, one of the preschool teacher's aides, thinks she's great with the kids but often spends her time cleaning and straightening instead of engaging the children. Harold, the other preschool teacher's aide, is quiet and mostly seems oblivious to what's around him, but the kids adore him. Stacey, the head preschool teacher, is their supervisor. She is a good teacher but often annoyed with her fellow staff members for not taking greater responsibility.

Marsha asked some clarifying questions but also wondered what it was like supervising them. Patricia admitted that she had found it difficult. She had only become director 2 years ago, but this staff had been here for many years except for Tyra. Since Patricia had taken over, everyone had improved, but it wasn't easy. Marsha reminded her that staffing issues were something they could talk about. Patricia rejected this, "You are really here for the kids. The adult problems are my responsibility." Marsha's attempt to expand her role was, at least initially, thwarted.

She tried a different tack, "Knowing some about the staff makes me feel so much more confident about meeting them. It makes me think of two other introductions that I think would be useful. Maybe I could spend some time telling the staff about myself and my hopes for consultation. Secondly, I wonder if the staff could give me a sense of the children?" This made sense to Patricia, and she agreed to, although still resisted, a group meeting. Marsha thought the group gathering would be important. In just the short description of staff, relationships seemed at the very least strained. She worried that if she met with one, someone would feel left out or targeted, "I know I am being a pest about this, but sometimes I meet with staff during nap time. Do you think that would be possible?" Patricia argued that there was no way that she could get all of the staff to meet at the same time—she had to consider coverage. Marsha asked if meeting separately with the preschool and toddler staff was any easier. Patricia could tolerate this compromise, and they scheduled the first set of meetings. Patricia identified the preschool as the place to begin, citing the preponderance of "special needs" children as the reason. Marsha ended by asking, "How was this meeting for you? I know you have reason to be leery, but does consultation seem any clearer or more likely to benefit your program?" Patricia surprised her, "This was great. I think that we have a plan, and I know that there are several kids who need your help." Aware that Patricia's trust in her return was likely fragile, Marsha offered to call to confirm the next visit. Patricia welcomed the reassurance.

As they came out of their meeting at 6:00 p.m., Tyra was nervously shuffling papers and did not look up. Marsha introduced herself as Tyra continued to occupy herself with the pile of forms. When Marsha explained what she was there for and their upcoming meeting, Tyra said "Good, the people I work with need help, especially Bob." "Well I hope that I can be helpful to everyone," Marsha replied carefully trying to avoid participating in slighting Bob.

Marsha realized that she hadn't finalized the hours that she would come, but Patricia seemed less concerned about that now. They had, however, scheduled two staff meetings over the next week. As she put her coat on to go, she realized that she could hear Patricia talking on the phone through the closed door. Looking up, she saw that the office was open at the rafters. Her conversation with Patricia had not been as confidential as she had thought.

Throughout this example, the consultant weighed the wish to respond to the director's immediate needs with the desire to appreciate the process and a stance of wondering. Marsha considered Patricia's willingness and ability to explore, her past consultation experiences, and perceptions. Marsha also acknowledged that the invitation to consult came from the director. As yet Marsha knew nothing of the staff's openness to or expectation of consultation. Although she was not able to discuss all of these issues directly, she had them in mind as she made choices about her responses. On her own and in supervision, she would follow these interactions by creating hypotheses—to be tested throughout consultation—about the meaning of Patricia's as well as her staff's reactions. Below we begin to address some of these issues while acknowledging that this discussion is certainly not exhaustive.

From the very beginning of this consultation scenario, Patricia's reluctance to begin seems to be related to the immediate experiences with the prior consultants, exacerbated by a general sensitivity to expected abandonment. As the consultation continues it will be important to watch for these reactions and to note the director's way of engaging new people. Patricia seemed to think that Marsha might take advantage of her, as indicated by her insistence on the amount of time. Individual interactions with the consultant alert us to a consultee's characteristic approach to other situations and relationships.

Consultants also have challenges that impact the way that they will perceive the process. Marsha initially interprets the director's protective pushing away and accusations of insufficiency as personal affronts. Luckily, Marsha quickly quells her anxiety and frustration. Rather than resting with her own assumptions of the director's behavior, she inquires about its meaning. Although Marsha is capable of acknowledging her own participation in the process, the outside help of a supervisor will guide her consideration of contributions to the many interactions inherent in consultation. For instance, Marsha's desire to make a broad difference (a common wish) may be thwarted by the beliefs and functioning of those involved. Marsha has yet to see the program in action, but she is already questioning how she will work with the two teachers that she met—Tyra and Leticia, both of whom immediately blame and belittle others in the program. Marsha suspects these teachers lack personal responsibility in their interactions. As Marsha collaborates with these teachers, she will have to balance her wish to affect change and her discomfort with individual's reactions with empathy for the individuals who most likely will only cooperate when experiencing general understanding and appreciation for their contributions. Despite the fact that she is not always patient with the children, Leticia needs to know her experiences as a parent are seen. Tyra's nervousness about how she is perceived may contribute to her criticizing her colleagues.

The consultant has demonstrated her willingness to consider their full experience. Marsha has indicated specifically her wish to be helpful in a number of arenas—parent–staff relationships, interstaff relationships, child–adult interactions, and program practices among others—but she has also demonstrated her approach through her behavior. Handling Patricia's repeated rejections, Marsha responded to Patricia with respect and a wish to understand her behavior.

Despite the fact that pushing new people away may be part of Patricia's personal style, even the most seasoned consultant occasionally blanches under repeated dismissals. As the consultant affords staff the experiences of being understood and gaining knowledge, the consulting agency should provide consultants with a similar forum. The supervisory relationship can offer a respite from the demands of consultation but also proffers a model for the consultant that can affect the consultation relationship. For instance, the supervisor's questioning, despite the consultant's initial frustration, allows Marsha to uncover truths. Because Marsha discovers Patricia's possible feelings of abandonment in Patricia's behavior, she develops a greater empathy for Patricia, resulting in patience and better targeted interventions. Consequently, Marsha will be able to tolerate the behavior directed toward her. Consultation succeeds through relationships and even the best consultant may have difficulty extracting herself from the process to objectively view the interactions. The consultant, like the child-care provider, needs an outside yet empathic eye.

The consultation process flows and ebbs. Hours of services usually vary at different parts of the year depending on the configuration of observation, staff meetings, and individual services. Marsha agrees to 5 hours, not because she thinks that a set amount of time ensures effectiveness or is always able to be used (most likely weekly hours of service will vary greatly), but because Patricia currently needs the reassurance of Marsha's commitment to be present.

Throughout, the consultant must construct the agenda with the provider. In this case, Patricia has ideas about how to use consultation—influenced, in part, by her anxiety about being cheated. Although the consultant is responsive to Patricia, she does not abandon her ideas. Marsha shares her view that staff meetings would be useful to better understand observations. However, she does not outwardly insist on staff meetings. Although a consultant might believe that regular meetings are the most effective way to bring about change, in some programs, staff meetings may not at least initially be possible. The consultant may need to hold this ideal and underline the importance of staff meetings without being adamant about them in the beginning.

A time for staff to talk with one another and with the consultant can be an aim of consultation. Holding fast to the belief that a forum for exchange is crucial to quality care, the consultant works to imbue this value to others but does not impose it. Only as the value of meeting is felt will a program internalize its importance and establish the practice.

This brings us to the boundaries of therapy and consultation—a delicate balance. The mental health professional's knowledge of human motivations, character structure, and defenses informs her understanding of and guides her interactions with the consultee. Marsha clearly sees some personal challenges that impede the process; Patricia's possible fear of abandonment affects her openness to consultation. She does not interpret this behavior in the moment and may never without the consent of Patricia. This does not mean, however, that she won't eventually, nor does it mean that she abandons this awareness. She underlines and responds to the feelings when possible. For instance, she comments on the challenges of abrupt good-byes for people in general assuming that this is also Patricia's distress. More subtly, Marsha commits to arriving 5 hours a week despite her belief that greater flexibility in time would be more beneficial in the long run; however, Patricia needs the reassurance that Marsha's agreement provides.

Understanding is the cornerstone of the therapeutic process. Throughout, Marsha was aware that her behavior would help to anticipate the course of consultation and telegraph her expectations and beliefs in mutual understanding. At several moments, she indicated her wish to understand the children, the staff, and the director and her plan to be respectful of each.

Assigned/Contracted

With the increase in attention and public funds for early childhood education and services, not all consultation is completely voluntary. Some consulting agencies and child-care programs have been assigned to each other. Initially, contracts that stipulate the length of service, the weekly amount of time, and the types and ratio of services provided may relieve some of the pressures of figuring out the particulars and each other, but there are limitations. Even child-care programs that request consultation ask to institute contracts to alleviate uncertainty and to create a sense of clarity. In any case, the circumstances need to be considered and addressed by the consultant with the child-care program. Although establishing parameters for consultation can be clarifying, rigidly adhering to an agreement that is defined before the needs of a program and its ability to use mental health consultation are known is usually problematic. Successful consultation relies on flexibility and adaptability to the shifting needs of a program.

When a third party initiates the match between consultant and consultee it may seem less voluntary. In these instances, the request is not necessarily based on an immediate or particular need of the child-care program. Despite the fact that this deviates from the voluntary basis of consultation, there are benefits as well as obstacles.

Embarking on consultation in the absence of crisis provides an unusual opportunity. The consultant and the program can establish familiarity without the pressure of a distressing situation needing resolution. This may promote more thoughtfulness as the program designs the combination of services right for them and identifies areas of concerns.

Drawbacks in this arrangement exist. One of the limitations is the recipients' loss of control or investment in the process. The loss of the power of choice—an important component of consultation—may be more keenly felt for providers who already feel at the mercy of low salaries, long hours, and demanding children and parents. In addition, programs that have identified a need for consultation are usually more open to services; therefore, establishing a working relationship may take longer in a setting where a consultant is assigned. One of the ways of establishing credibility and the tone of consultation was by responsiveness through the initial negotiation. This form of modeling is no longer available through the negotiation process. Third, because the impetus for service is no longer a defined problem, where to begin becomes less clear. The consultant and program will need to work hard to find focus, establish need, and create investment.

A contract assumes a level of agreement not yet established. The language and the meaning of the particulars may not be universally understood or interpreted, leading to misunderstandings. Even programs not required to establish and to fulfill contracts may attempt to codify their relationship. The contract may alleviate the anxiety of entering a new, not yet understood process; however, even when created together the language will be understood differently as the consultant and the child-care program come from different perspectives and have distinct areas of professional focus (mental health and early childhood education).

Therefore, establishing the parameters of the consultation relationship and the services remains crucial despite the contractual support for the particulars. The safety of the contract will tempt new consultants as well as child-care directors to rely solely on the written word to establish roles. However, consultation is a process; therefore, the consultant must address the wishes and interpretations of the staff in the beginning as well as throughout the process. The contract offers a limited two-dimensional description of consultation, a living, growing process. Relying solely on the contractual agreement will stunt the process, in part, because participants are agreeing to a broad set of services that are difficult to understand before and even while experiencing them.

As consultees become more comfortable with services, they will be open to expanded definitions that uncertainty may have preempted. For instance, how can one describe the consultant's willingness to address the individual caregivers' life histories and challenges as they impact the work with children? Rarely have child-care providers in the initial stages of consultation assumed this connection, or more importantly, been willing to share this level of intimacy. Yet, we believe that this becomes one of the most important aspects of transforming child-care relationships. Solidifying the arrangement prior to consultation and referring solely to the original agreement can handicap the organic development.

Matching the Consultant

Information gathered in the request for consultation is considered in the consultant assignment. The agency providing consultation is not always able to pick from a plethora of candidates, but when possible consultant characteristics should be considered. It is fortunate when a consultation agency has the opportunity to assign someone who most meets the needs of the requesting child-care program. For instance, a director who is calling because her staff just can't get along may benefit from a consultant with more experience with adult group dynamics. Yet, some programs struggle as they attempt to establish developmentally appropriate curriculum and would benefit from a consultant with a background in early childhood education. In other instances, personal characteristics influence the choice of consultant. A program composed of seasoned veterans who are wary of outside assistance may be best matched with an older, more mature consultant or at least one who exudes an old-shoe ease and can more confidently manage the lack of enthusiasm for her presence.

Although not entirely possible due to the varied ethnic make-up of each child care and the ethnicities of available consultants, efforts should be made to match programs with a consultant who represents the cultural background of the programs constituency, both providers and family. Of course, ethnicity is only one area of people's experience, but sameness, real or perceived, can foster trust more easily in the initial stages. Finally, every effort must be made to match those with language capabilities beyond English to programs with large non-English speaking populations. Linguistic limitations can, obviously, preclude consultation from occurring. Therefore, language capacity is a primary consideration in assigning consultants. However, here again, many languages may be spoken in a single center. (Consultants actively and thoughtfully engage translators as needed.)

During the initial request, the intake coordinator should cull and consider a program's consultant preferences. Understanding the ethnic and linguistic make-up of the staff and children begins this process. A full understanding of the needs of a program and the working style of the participants will also lead to a good match. Every consultant addresses myriad and diverse issues. Therefore, all must be prepared to deal with the range of consultative situations from the individual child to broad programmatic concerns. As usual however, not all can be anticipated and even the seemingly best match can become a challenge. No matter how well planned, every consultant will have to address misunderstandings, and misperceptions. For instance, an African-American consultant matched with a primarily African-American program may be initially greeted with more acceptance than her Caucasian counterpart, but her level of education and economic status might breed its own form of resentment requiring exploration later in the process.

Summary

As many children are reminded by their mother on their way to their first day of school, first impressions really are important. Consultation is a relationship process that begins at the initial request. The way in which the consultant and her agency respond to the expressed need will influence the ongoing relationship and its effectiveness. As the new consultant begins, she must look at the interactions closely to discover the meaning of behavior.

The ways in which she engages the staff telegraphs both her regard and respect for their relationship as it begins and her approach to understanding and helping children. Consultation is a collaborative effort. She values the contribution of all participants, hopes to understand and voice the subjective experience of the children as well as the adults, and expects to consider and explore behavior before reacting. She needs to understand the staff's expectations, assess their investment, gather their understanding of the challenges that are faced, and agree upon strategies.

Every child-care program has a different configuration of adults contributing to the care of children. Their varied levels of expertise, perceptions, approaches, and personal histories will all influence the consultation. The consultant attempts to identify these contributors as they arise. In addition, the way in which a program begins consultation will also affect the process. We addressed three modes: the director- or staff-initiated request, the transfer of consultant, and the assigned or contracted consultation arranged by a third party. Each offers particular opportunities and impediments. Bread and Jam Child Care was introduced as a program having previously received consultation that was recently assigned a new consultant. We will follow this program throughout subsequent chapters as we attempt to delineate the consultation process.

Finally, although we hope that any consultant will be able to establish a relationship with a particular program, we know that matching consultants can initially make the process easier. The parameters for pairing a consultant to a program may include some combination of her particular area of expertise, her ethnicity or cultural experience, her linguistic capacities, and her confidence level, among others. Of course, the efficacy of these initial matches will be redefined as the consultant and her consultees come to know each other. Consultation always values the experience of the participants.

Chapter 3

Getting to Know the Program

In our discussion of initiating consultation, we began to formulate ideas about how a child-care program functions and understands itself and the children. This chapter continues that focus as the consultant's discovery deepens. The process of "getting to know" is ongoing for child-care programs are ever-changing entities. Therefore, the phase of learning about a program may last a few months to a year as the consultant meets the various participants. Sometimes that process begins again—a consultant may add a new classroom to her workload, new staff members may join the program, or the composition of the children shifts, changing the balance of consultation. Ultimately, the process is always dynamic.

Getting to Know Whom?

As described in the previous chapter, consultees often begin by asking the consultant to "get to know" a specific child who may be signaling difficulty. Whether the request is child specific or programmatic, the efforts remain the same. In order to help a child, the consultant must identify the lens through which caregivers are examining the child. Whether she is getting to know a child or caregiver, the consultant's stance is unchanging—she wonders with the participants about the part each plays in the situation toward developing a mutually held understanding of difficulties and solutions.

In this chapter, we will attempt to understand a program—its staff and its children—by examining the expectations of caregivers, the program's philosophy of child care and child development, the organizational structure with its associated roles and relationships, and the individuals who compose the program. Even as caregivers focus on particular children, the consultant is creating opportunities to understand as much as possible about all aspects of the child-care community. Methods for fostering those opportunities include direct questioning; observation; wondering how providers make choices and decisions; establishing relationships; and formulating, testing, and reconceptualizing hypotheses about behavior.

Finally, the successful consultant straddles the line between the role of participant in the relationships that create change in a child-care program and that of an objective observer who hopes to understand a program's participants, free from the constraints of that program's hierarchy and functioning. For example, the consultant may rely on the goodwill of one of the staff members who is particularly open to her presence. Her comfortable relationship with the staff member may allow inquiries of a personal nature that facilitate discovery of the individual's contribution to and understanding of the problem and program. This special relationship may also foster implementation of interventions with children. At the same time, however, others are observing the interactions between the consultant and the staff member and their relationship. A staff member who resents this "special relationship" or feels excluded will undoubtedly act out these feelings with the consultant or even with her coworker—possibly destabilizing existing relationships in the program. The consultant must be able to observe her impact on all participants in the program—balancing her wish for closeness and its benefits with the effect of her behavior on others who are not as accepting or available to consultation.

This chapter focuses on how questions about and the experience of a child offer insight into a program's functioning and understanding of itself. The child may be the impetus for conversation, but the consultant's focus remains on how the providers have come to know that child. How they understand the child says as much about the program—its functioning and its philosophy—as it does about the child. For now, we will leave concentration on the child for later chapters with the understanding that case consultation and programmatic consultation are necessarily intertwined. However, the understanding of the child always reveals caregivers' perceptions of children in general and of themselves. For the moment, we will consider children only as a way of understanding the culture of a program. In actual consultation, we address child and program issues simultaneously.

What to Know? Attempting to Understand

Chapter 2 introduced the idea that consultation happens directly and indirectly. The consultant needs to be aware of both explicit and implicit communication—a process that becomes easier as information is culled through observation, direct questioning, and interactions. With each layer of information, the consultant develops new interpretations and uses them in interventions. The responses to those interventions add new dimensions and complexity to the overall understanding and affect future interactions.

Although information can be harvested in a number of ways, which will be discussed later, the fruits remain the same. These are expectations and perceptions of the consultant and each other, the philosophy of care, the organizational structure, roles and relationships, and the idiosyncrasies of individuals. The subjects we have picked are crucial for understanding a program and the perceptions of its individual members, but this list is not exhaustive. Of course, each source of information grows and changes and therefore needs constant tending and examination.

Expectations and Perceptions

As discussed in chapter 2, providers will have expectations of the consultant that range from the ineffective and useless to the heroic and miraculous. Most likely, the consultant's capacities fall somewhere in between. In the initial stages of their relationship, the consultant asks providers about their previous experience and understanding of consultation. Descriptions of prior use of consultation will reveal the providers' openness to the experience as well as to the possibility of success. As providers come to know the consultant, expectations shift. Even those caregivers who have had positive experiences with previous consultants may be wary of the new one. Sometimes a program's past experience engenders positive institutional transference. The new consultant can ride the wave of goodwill established by her predecessor. However, positive expectations can intimidate a consultant who feels that she cannot live up to them.

Expectations are not restricted to the apparent efficacy of the consultant's contributions. Practical aspects of consultation are also anticipated and based on past experiences. For example, a teacher who is told that the consultant is there to "help" may expect her to watch over the classroom while the teacher takes her break. Another hears that the consultant will "assist" with a particularly difficult child and becomes disappointed when she discovers the child will not be seen in individual therapy outside the classroom. The consultant must identify these wishes in questions, requests, and complaints as well as in the providers' behaviors.

Although one might assume that speakers of a common language understand its words in the same way, in fact people imbue words with meaning not only according to their formal definition but also according to the speaker's and listener's histories—personal and cultural. (This is true for all native English speakers but becomes even more complicated as English-as-a-second-language speakers are considered.) As always, the consultant should *wonder* about, rather than assume, a provider's view.

Perhaps most important to our thesis that relationships form the cornerstone of consultation is the idea that someone's expectations of the consulting relationship express that person's internal experience of relationships in general. For example, the teacher who, like some of her students, grew up in a neglectful home, may come to see the consultant's attempts to be objective as discounting. In response to feeling again overlooked, the provider employs familiar ways of coping. She may withdraw from the consultant, inadvertently confirming her own expectation of neglect. Alternately, a provider whose life experiences cause her to see attention as synonymous with scrutiny interprets the consultant's inquiry as intrusive. As in the process of therapy, the mental health consultant's position as both an outsider and possible authority figure creates a screen for projection of inner conflicts and individuals' expectations of relationships. In her interactions, the consultant is making and testing hypotheses and watching for and asking about providers' reactions. Uncovering these processes is a crucial step toward making effective connections between the provider and consultant. Furthermore, providers' views of relationships often reveal their understanding and approach to relationships with children. Therefore, the consultant identifies participants' expectations of her role as well as their expectations of the relationship—not only to create an effective consultation relationship but also, and equally essential, to understand the caregivers' approach to others and, ultimately, to children.

The consultant's relationship to each provider offers a powerful illustration of these dynamics, but not the only one. The providers' expectations of each other also reveal crucial information. The consultant can confirm or challenge her assumptions about their relationship styles by observing the providers' relationships with each other and comparing and contrasting them to her experience with each of them. Sometimes a provider has the ability to foster wonderful relationships with children while struggling with her colleagues, but, most often, the regard she has for her coworkers predicts her interactions with children. Of course, the comparison is easily made because staff relationships and teacher–child relationships are immediately observable. Observation of adult relationships often facilitates interpretation of staff–child relationships. A caregiver who dismisses her coworkers' offers of assistance and yet constantly complains about being unsupported indicates her sense that relationships are not reciprocal. This view likely extends to her behavior with children. She demands autonomy and ignores children's bids for help. Her stance toward coworkers and children is rooted in her own experience of the world. Perhaps a history of disrupted relationships solidified a world view that renounces needs and exalts independence to protect against an overwhelming fear that her unmet dependency needs will be discounted.

Philosophy of Care

The consultant asks about and attempts to understand each program's guiding philosophy. A program's philosophy, combined with providers' expectations and ideas of child rearing and development, informs program practices. The consultant's contributions must be tailored to the program's views of the child-care landscape.

The philosophy of care offers context for the consultant's observations, interpretations, and interventions. The needs of children ultimately dictate the functioning of child care, but the interpreted needs of the children—whether academic or emotional—will determine the explanations for and language surrounding the program's practices. Most programs, for example, will have circle time, but the reasons given for including it will vary: One program will describe it as an organized opportunity for teaching concepts and self-control; another will speak of it as a time for social exchange and interaction. Both philosophies have benefits, but providers will lean toward or value one purpose more than others. Knowing what the program values helps the consultant find language to discuss challenges and foster the provider's investment. In a program wedded to teaching preacademic skills, a consultant espouses, in vain, the usefulness of following a daily schedule until she endows the schedule with the power to prepare children for the rigors of kindergarten. Conversely, underlining the importance of anticipating transitions is a congenial fit for a program that sees social–emotional development as primary.

Organizational Structure

Most child-care programs have some delineated hierarchy. The chain of command can serve as a map to the consultant navigating the most effective routes for intervention. The consultant must assess the lines of hierarchy, the intensity of adherence to these guidelines, and how they affect consultation. A director who prides herself on running a tight ship expects that every step the consultant takes be cleared through her. Another director who feels overwhelmed by her role excludes herself from consultant–staff contact, hoping the consultant can relieve her of responsibilities. Alternately, a program that operates on consensus building involves everyone equally in the meetings.

The way that individual positions are described suggests their inherent value. Are there head teachers, teachers, and aides? How many levels of supervision exist—a director, site supervisor, head teacher, teacher, and assistants? How fluidly can members at different levels communicate with each other? In addition to the formal hierarchy, patterns of communication among staff set the stage for the consultant's entrance. For example, well-established staff meetings make it easier for the consultant to create change, but in some programs staff communicate with each other only through informal exchanges on the fly. A program's forums for communication indicate the value it places on input from various staff members and negotiation among them.

A program's expressed organizational structure may vary from what is actually practiced or wished for. Here again, the experiences and psychologies of individuals will influence the program's functioning and, by association, its receptiveness to the consultant.

Roles and Relationships

Its organizational structure offers a framework for approaching a program, yet how participating adults actually function in and interpret the role of "teacher" or "aide" varies greatly from program to program. In addition to their assigned jobs, members of a team accept and act out roles. In one program, the older assistant teacher who takes great pride in her role as the matriarch of her family brings that same confidence to the classroom, becoming the leader to whom the young head teacher looks for approval. Although the consultant should be constantly studying these dynamics, the participants will have their own analyses. Understanding the providers' definitions of their roles and responsibilities is most important.

Their relationships inside and outside the child-care setting affect providers' functioning in their roles. Only after she has wondered about the functioning of a child's family member, for example, may a consultant discover that one of the teachers is the child's cousin or aunt. Within a child-care program, members may be related, enacting their family dynamics in the child-care setting without revealing the connection. Often, others feel excluded without fully understanding the reasons.

Sometimes members of a program will form preferential relationships that exclude other staff members or that favor a particular family. Similarly, parents in a program may naturally gravitate to the teacher who most closely resembles them in ethnicity, experiences, or economic status, subverting the formal channels of communication. In one program, the staff and consultant determined that a family's well-being would be better protected if a child's poor behavior wasn't reported every evening at pick-up. All supposedly agreed that a particular teacher would present "bad news" if necessary but that all would make an effort to share positive aspects of the child's day. The teacher's assistant, however, had already created a special relationship with the child's family. She braided family members' hair for a fee, she attended the children's birthday parties with her own children, and she saw the family in her neighborhood. To hold back information when asked directly felt like a betrayal of this family with whom she had become close, and she feared that revealing the dual relationship might jeopardize her job—especially since she had been warned against forming business relationships with families. The family's and the assistant teacher's wishes to help each other out, based on their shared economic status and culture, had superceded the decisions of the classroom, but initially no one else was aware of what had happened. These exclusive connections affect staff relationships, and other parents and children will also wonder about, perhaps resent, or compete for priority status.

Individual Providers

From the moment the consultant enters the program, she and the providers are sizing each other up. The consultant slowly learns about various personalities in the program and how they relate to each other and to her. As she interacts with staff members, she considers their idiosyncrasies. More important, she learns about the reasons underlying these traits so that she can best tailor her responses to each individual.

Consider the teacher who seems to display little warmth toward the children for fear of "spoiling" them and responds with less than lukewarm enthusiasm to suggestions for creating time for individual interaction with each child. Nothing seems to shift until the consultant begins to unearth information about the teacher's experience of early deprivation and her resulting withdrawal from intimate interaction. A deeper understanding often allows the consultant to construct her suggestions in ways that approach the caregiver's underlying wish for empathy and offer a corrective experience of relationships. The consultant's exploration and actions are intended to be therapeutic, but the consultation relationship is distinct from psychotherapy.

How One Knows: Gathering Information

We have suggested that there are numerous relationships, structures, and perceptions of which the consultant should be aware, but orienting oneself in this thicket of information can be challenging. How does the consultant actually begin to explore? The following suggestions may seem obvious, but new consultants forget these concepts initially. Even the most seasoned consultants step away from the first few weeks in a new program wondering what they should have done and where they are headed. Ultimately, you are creating opportunities to expose the path and the obstacles that you must avoid as you move toward your destination—helping programs function better. Below, we offer equipment that you will need on the journey.

Direct Questioning

Never underestimate the effectiveness of the direct question. Consultants sometimes feel that direct questions are too intrusive. But scheduling and resource constraints often limit the time a consultant can spend with staff. Asking people about their experience, their decisions, and their understanding can offer quick clarification, reduce misunderstandings, and foster honest, straightforward exchanges that promote trust in the consultation relationship. The intent is to convey interest, not accusation. How one asks differentiates the two.

Directness can be confounded with aggressiveness. This need not be the case if the tone of the question is inclusive and wondering. Direct questions can also be open-ended. The difference between "Why did you do that?" and "How did you make that decision?" is great, despite the same underlying wish to understand choices made. The answer to "how" questions will reveal the facts as well as the thinking process. A question beginning with "why" will often receive a defensively short response.

Observation Accompanied by Questioning

Observation affords another avenue for getting to know a program. There are various types of and purposes for observing: (a) classroom and child observations that include teacher–child interactions; (b) observations of adult relationships and interactions; and (c) observations of individual adults and their interactions with the consultant. This chapter focuses on adults and their relationship to one another. The consultant's initial observations require agreement and permission but also require a certain level of focus and understanding of the program prior to beginning (to be discussed in further detail in the chapter on observation of children). These prior pieces of information might include classroom schedules and management as well as teacher–child relationships. Observation of adults offers insight into the areas addressed in this chapter.

The consultant can observe adults in staff meetings, adult interactions within the classroom, adults' descriptions of each other, and their ways of interacting with the consultant. Every moment that a consultant spends in a child-care program should involve observation. Observation is an awareness of all components of a program's functioning. Prior assessments and theories bring focus and direction to observations designed to confirm or refute those theories. The consultant's interpretation of her observations directs her to new areas or depths of exploration.

Tentative Hypotheses and Formulations

As she observes, the consultant constantly seeks to understand the meaning of the behavior she sees and form tentative hypotheses and formulations that are open to expansion. Interpretations focus observation. Hypotheses require testing, and the effective consultant evaluates them through her observations, questions, and interactions.

Relationship

Each member of the team forms a unique relationship to the consultant. These relationships vary in depth and closeness, but each offers indispensable data. How people value and use relationships indicates their ability to work with each other and with the children. The consultant must find ways to be useful and responsive to each member of the team (some participants make this infinitely easier than others). Individual differences can be a trap for the consultant, who will naturally gravitate toward staff members who are responsive. Yet successful interventions depend on working with the entire system; the consultant must pay attention to each relationship.

How One Stands: The Consultant's Positioning

Before the consultant arrives, and between visits, the program operates on its own—filling gaps and making do. In the day-to-day life of the program, as well as in the beginning of the consultation relationship, the consultant has to insert herself into a running drama. The roles she accepts will influence the receptivity of the providers, affect the ongoing consultation process, and start to establish the providers' expectations for her work. These responses to the consultant's role work in conjunction and against each other as the consultant orients herself.

Because her presence can be imbued with powerful hopes, the consultant must enter gingerly. Expanding involvement over time is easier than eliminating established expectations. Consequently, the consultant must not immediately accept a major part in the program's functioning. Restraint can be a challenge in a beleaguered system where providers are begging the consultant to contribute. Circumstances and the providers' wishes will pull the consultant to jump into action in the classroom. The caregivers will initially welcome the extra hands and the consultant will feel immediately effective. A consultant must resist this pull for several reasons: (a) Being hands-on creates expectations that ultimately disappoint providers because this role will not always be possible or successful; (b) while "doing" helps providers in the moment, it is not instructive; (c) acting can inadvertently communicate a sense of being more skillful than the provider; and (d) action forfeits the future advantages of being able to observe from outside the system.

Straddling the line between participant and observer allows the consultant to make sense of the relationships and roles in the program. Abandoning the participant–observer stance makes it impossible to assess the hierarchies and relationships among the providers. By entering the program as an extra set of hands, yet with the special status of a knowledgeable outsider who most likely intimidates the others, the consultant immediately and irreversibly alters the system without the benefit of preliminary observations from which to chart systemic changes. However, standing outside the system, the consultant is neither limited by its restrictions nor embedded in its hierarchies. In one program, for example, a misinterpretation of the practice of redirecting children led the teachers to believe that they could never say no to children. When the consultant intervened with a child by firmly telling him no, she violated the rule and used a tool not available to the others. The teachers resented her freedom, but her role as the expert prevented them from questioning her. Instead, they felt misunderstood—and they were. The consultant assumed that their reluctance to contain the children resulted from their personal limitations rather than the limits of the perceived practice. Watching interactions with children and wondering with the teachers later would have been more useful and instructive for the caregivers and the consultant.

The consultant's consistent message to providers is that people notice and make meaning of what you do. This principle holds true when a consultant takes a hands-on role in a classroom. Although some staff will find the consultant's stepping in helpful, others may interpret her action as an indictment of their failure in the classroom—not to mention the feelings arising from the apparent success (or lack of) of the consultant's interventions. Of course, the outside-observer stance can be interpreted as aloof or unhelpful, yet we have found that it is ultimately the safer place to begin. Preparing providers and explaining the reasons for the consultant's positioning can alleviate some of the drawbacks of the outside-observer stance.

Ultimately, the initiating phase of consultation creates opportunities to learn about the child-care community. The best position for doing so usually is located slightly outside the scene: The consultant is able to jump in when absolutely necessary but is far enough back so that true observation is possible. Once the consultant is ensconced in the setting, she can no longer get a full view. Furthermore, any entrance irreparably alters the system.

Case Example

Holding in mind the consultant's considerations in getting to know a program, we return to Bread and Jam Child Care. The consultant, Marsha, arrives for her arranged meeting with the preschool staff. The little boy, Leo, who was alluded to in the consultant's first visits, quickly comes to the fore. While acknowledging the staff's wish for case consultation, the consultant maintains the fuller focus of familiarizing herself with the program. At this point in consultation, focusing on a particular child may be safer for the teachers and directly addressing their concerns without unduly escalating anxiety by requiring immediate self-reflection. For the moment, the consultant holds the role of reflection while she looks for opportunities to give information about consultation and learn about the individuals and system in which she will immerse herself. She frames her questions with the underlying intent of understanding programmatic issues. She thinks constantly about what her interactions, observations, and direct questioning reveal about the program's functioning, weaving the concerns about a child into a broader context. She is also careful to consider and clarify expectations about her role. We rejoin the consultant in her efforts at "getting to know."

> Marsha arrived early for her first naptime meeting with the preschool staff because she wanted to review the agenda with the director. Patricia was missing in action. The school secretary, Rosie, informed her that Patricia may have forgotten about the meeting and added, "I hadn't been told about it which means it's not going to happen." Rosie then wanted to know why the consultant was there before she would track Patricia down. She asked Marsha questions about her education, and her marital status and inquired about children. Marsha struggled with her own impatience and responded. After reviewing Marsha's qualifications, Rosie tracked Patricia down on the intercom. Patricia had forgotten but would be there shortly. While waiting together Rosie continued, "So you must be meeting with the preschool room. They have a kid in there who can't be controlled. He's in the office every other day, but I can get him in line. I just tell him to go sit over there and give him dirty looks until he stops. Then I usually give him some candy. I'm not sure what's going on in that classroom. My daughter tells me that he is always in trouble." Rosie didn't seem old enough to have an adult daughter. Marsha would discover much later that Rosie was referring to her 4-year-old daughter. She continued, "Besides you'll be glad not to meet with the toddler teachers. They never get along." Marsha noted the view of inter-staff conflict but directed her response to Rosie's experience, "You seem to know everything that's going on here." Rosie smiled proudly, revealing that she had been here longer than most of the staff and knew more than anyone about the families.

In this brief interaction, Marsha can begin to form hypotheses about the hierarchy and the functioning of the agency. As in many programs, the secretary has a position that belies her role of administrative support. Self-appointed or generally accepted, Rosie's place in the school's functioning will figure into the consultant's success. Because she is not a member of the teaching staff, she will not likely participate in meetings, and yet her power may influence functioning.

Patricia came in with Leo. He was kicking and screaming as she dragged him in. She put him in a chair across from Rosie. Rosie looked harshly at him, and just as she said, he quieted down. He cried quietly in the corner, and Marsha resisted comforting him. Spying Marsha, Patricia gasped with exasperation, "Oh, right, we're meeting with the preschool staff. Just go in the room, I'll join you as soon as I can." Marsha shared her wish to meet prior to their meeting with the staff. Patricia wasn't so sure.

Appreciating the pulls on Patricia's time, Marsha bargained for a few minutes. Patricia pointed to Leo, "There's our topic for today." Marsha understood the urgency but also wanted to use the meeting to get to know the staff. She again felt like she was struggling with slowing down, but reassurances that she remembered the wish to focus on Leo soothed Patricia. First, Marsha needed to get to know the staff and the center in order to understand the child. She clarified before the group assembled—Patricia would lead the meeting, introduce Marsha, and the teachers would introduce themselves and their program—all within 45 minutes.

Marsha must quickly interpret Patricia's tardiness. Combining Patricia's defensive disengagement with the possibility of an extensive workload, Marsha responds to both, showing respect for Patricia's time and reassuring her that her concerns will be addressed. Marsha does not give up her wish to meet and understand the staff and their relationships. Instead, she blends her wish with Patricia's concerns; understanding Leo gives Patricia an incentive for meeting as a group.

The meeting should have begun by now, but Marsha sat by herself. Finally, Leticia, the teacher's aide, who had met Marsha on the yard a couple of weeks ago straggled in with a cup of coffee, "That was a long morning. I thought we were supposed to meet today?" Marsha concurred and thanked Leticia for remembering. Leticia left Marsha alone to round up the other people. She then heard an announcement from Rosie over the intercom for the staff to assemble. After 15 minutes, the final staff member—Patricia—entered. Marsha wondered if she should start without her given the teaching staff was present but maintained the agreement that she and the director had established. Informally chatting, she had already discovered that the staff seemed overwhelmed. Stacey, the head teacher, expressed resentment at waiting and meeting as she had other things to do for which she didn't have time. Leticia was just happy to have a break (although Stacey clarified exasperatedly, "She takes plenty of breaks…"). Other than greeting the consultant, Harold, another aide in the classroom, had not spoken, nor would he until close to the end of the meeting. In fact, he sat outside the circle of chairs Marsha had put together. Despite her invitation to join the circle, Harold kept his distance.

Veering from their agenda, Patricia introduced Marsha, "She is going to be here to fix Leo." Seeing the staff's excitement and fearing their ambitious expectations, Marsha shuddered but quickly recovered, saying, "That's true, I would like to help, but I think before we can attend to your concerns about Leo I will need to know something about the world in which he is struggling. I need to know you and your program. Besides, you and his parents know him best. I have to have some of the same information as you. I'm also aware that we have limited time today. Perhaps we could start with introductions. I would also like to hear about your past experiences with consultants and what was useful."

Stacey began, "I guess I should start since I'm the head teacher." Marsha couldn't be sure, but Leticia seemed to roll her eyes. Harold didn't engage at all. Stacey talked proudly of being a parent and of her education—a BA degree in child development. She described the previous consultant as helpful. When Marsha asked what in particular had been useful, Stacey spoke of the consultant's instructions to the other staff members. Stacey seemed determined to establish her personal lack of need for consultation and her staff's utter need for improvement. She then wondered about Marsha's age and experience, "You seem awfully young."

"I guess I am young when you consider all the experience you have had. You and the others are probably wondering what I could offer when you have so many years on me." Marsha stopped to query the others and marvel at their years of service to children. Stacey had been teaching for 15 years, and Leticia (60 years old) and Harold (55 years old) had been child-care workers for 25 and 18 years, respectively. Marsha had just turned 30—very young compared to everyone else. "There is so much knowledge in those years of experience with which I couldn't possibly compete. The good thing is that consultation relies on cooperation and not competition. I hope to add my understanding of young children to yours. I will have the opportunity and luxury to watch what happens here from outside your intensely demanding roles. I can offer observations and maybe ask the right questions to further our thinking about a child or your program. My experience has been with young children and their parents who are having difficulties; perhaps I could help with that too." Marsha talked a bit about her years of experience working in various mental health agencies and her familiarity with community resources.

Staff relationships, self-perceptions, and needs are beginning to emerge. Marsha notices but does not yet begin to comment or do anything about them. The staff expressed their initial perceptions of Marsha, revealing their hopes as well as their reservations. Stacey's desperation for respect for her role suggests a lack of confidence, which she attempts to cast on Marsha by questioning her age. Marsha does not shy away or become defensive; instead, she uses the opportunity to address the head teacher's worries. Here, she manages to straddle the roles of participant and observer. By embracing the staff's years of experience, the consultant shows respect for them and their reservations but creates an additional place for her role. She can do this because as an outsider she considers their questions and reactions as expressions of their own struggles, experiences, and goals.

In response to the consultant's description of her past experience working directly with parents and children, Leticia exclaims, "Oh great, because Leo really needs someone to work with him. We could use the extra help in the room." Marsha wonders, "Is that what previous consultants did?" It turns out that although the program had had a one-on-one aide for an individual child in the past, the previous consultant had not worked directly with children. Marsha recognized the request as an expression of the group's feeling overwhelmed, "I can sure understand your wish for immediate relief, but I worry that without knowing anything about him or your program my involvement on any level would interfere rather than help. Perhaps if I observed your classroom, I would have a better sense of your experience with him." When Marsha asked them on what she should focus, they all agreed Leo. She wondered therefore how they understood his difficulties and what conversations they had had with his mother. Actually, they had thought about neither. Marsha agreed to observe the classroom but voiced her reluctance to focus on Leo until his parents were aware of her involvement with the center. Leticia immediately complained that Leo's mother doesn't even say hello when she drops off Leo. "It sounds like she's not sure how to connect to the classroom. Maybe we can think about how to involve her in consultation and with all of you. We'll work on including her." Everyone seemed content, yet Harold remained quiet. With Marsha's prompting, Harold theorized, "Leo needs a man in his life." Marsha wondered what contributed to Harold's hypothesis. Harold concisely commented on his success in interacting with Leo. Everyone confirmed this view. Harold stayed silent for the remainder of the meeting, but when he left he smiled at Marsha and said, "Nice meeting."

Marsha manages two things. She holds the idea that parent involvement is important without dismissing the staff's frustrations, and she attends to the individuals' experience of her and each other. Marsha offers to initiate consultation around Leo, yet she voices her preference as to how the process proceeds. Considering providers' wishes and feelings need not mean abandoning the consultant's integrity. In the most ideal situations, the consultant can remain neutral while offering additional ideas for consideration, but sometimes providers feel too overwhelmed to contemplate the feelings of others or alternate solutions. When this is the case, the consultant can voice the other's subjective experience and sometimes offer her opinion. She subtly suggests that Leo's mother may not feel welcome—an explanation for her behavior that the staff has probably not considered. She also signals her expectation that Leo's mother be included in any consultation about Leo. With Harold, as well as the others, she watches for clues to reveal their involvement and investment with the children and the process of consultation. Marsha notices Harold hovering on the periphery and wonders whether this is an expression of his perceived outside status. She tests her hypothesis by eliciting his contribution and underscoring his relationship with Leo. Her obvious respect for his input allows him to briefly join the group. Whether or not she gives voice to what she observes, the consultant is always identifying and responding to the subjective experience of all participants.

> Marsha didn't want to end the first meeting without stating the obvious. She and Patricia were the only Caucasians in the room. "Along the way we are going to notice differences among us and between us and the children. We've already noticed age and experience. There will also be differences in the way that we were raised, our culture, our economic experiences, and education that affect the ways that we think and think about each other. One of the differences that is immediately apparent is ethnicity—and although it would most likely be difficult to talk about or even know how it will affect our interactions—I want to encourage you to let me know if my way of understanding any of you or the children and families you work with differs from your view. While I would hope not to misinterpret you or the children, our different experiences likely lead us to view the world in varying ways. I'll hope that you can tell me if you think I've gotten it wrong in some way." The group seems surprised.

Bringing attention to the subjective experience of all requires that undercurrents come to—and sometimes be nudged to—the surface. Cultural and ethnic differences are easily observed and bring a range of assumptions and judgments, but people usually avoid talking about them for fear of offending. By asserting early in the process that perception is determined by past experience, the consultant displays her ability and her wish to consider differing perspectives. To start where there are widely identified differences and likely unexpressed feelings and possible resentment shows Marsha's openness. In doing so the consultant conveys something about herself, but more important, she demonstrates the possibility for others to embrace differences and communicate without judgment.

> Stacey caught Marsha on the way out. Referring to her coworkers, she added, "Those two really need someone to tell them what to do. If I wasn't here, nothing would get done." Marsha commented on the amount of pressure Stacey must feel. She offered to meet with Stacey if she wanted, but the invitation was rejected.

Again, Marsha juggles the wish to be individually responsive with the need to support group cohesion. This parallel experience to the child-care setting offers opportunity for the consultant to practice these skills and build empathy for teachers who must corral 20 children while being responsive to each. With this interaction, Marsha is also building a formulation of the head teacher's personality and her needs. Stacey requests special recognition for her hard work and her role yet rejects individual attention when offered. Marsha will now watch for this theme in their interactions and Stacey's work.

> As she had agreed to, Marsha returned the following week to observe the classroom as a way of beginning to familiarize herself with the program's philosophy and routines as well as with the staff and children. She entered the classroom early in the morning. Most of the children had already arrived. She had discussed beforehand her introduction to parents—a person who was here to help the staff think about how the center could best serve all the children—and Patricia had sent a letter to the parents describing the new consultant as an addition to the team. Because Marsha was sitting near the door, she was able to introduce herself to parents as they came in. She noted that she was the only one greeting parents. Leo and his mother were struggling as they entered. He seemed sort of agitated as was his mother who was trying to sign in and leave quickly. Marsha tried to stop her to introduce herself, and Leo's mother said, "I am already late for work, and I don't have time to hear about how bad Leo was yesterday." Marsha responded,

"I'm sorry, I didn't mean to make a hectic time tougher, and I don't want to make you late. I just wanted to introduce myself as the new consultant and let you know that I'll be here from time to time to observe the classroom and meet with the teachers to help them create the best experience for each child. I am also available to parents when questions or concerns come up." She seemed relieved and excused herself. Marsha noticed that Mom and Leo had not said good-bye and that she was the only one who had greeted either of them. The consultant wondered if her presence had changed the routine at all.

This is the consultant's first program observation. Remembering her role as a participant–observer, Marsha watches with intent interest from a respectful remove. She is careful not to assume that this single observation represents the daily routine of the classroom. In addition, her presence may have already altered the interactions. While presenting herself to all the parents, she purposely engages the mother of the child on whom the staff wants to focus. Her interactions with Leo's mother confirm and refute the staff's preconceptions of her. Leo's mom rejects Marsha but warms with the reassurance that she will not be bombarded with bad news about her son. This parent's initial response alerts the consultant to her expectations, based likely on previous experiences with the teachers. Marsha doesn't push more for two reasons. Leo's mother may not be able to tolerate more, and Marsha doesn't want to usurp the teaching staff's role with respect to this or any other parent.

There were 22 children in the class and most of them were playing in small groups throughout the room. Although the consultant carefully avoids prolonged attention to Leo, she watches what he elicits in the providers. With his thumb in his mouth, Leo wandered to each group and observed briefly from the outskirts before moving on to the next group. His behavior surprised her because she had expected him to be disruptive. He went over to Leticia and watched her cut paper towels in two with scissors creating a large pile to sit next to the sink. She said hello as he leaned up against her but did not engage him further. He left her and circled around the classroom again. He lingered at the block area for a few minutes and pulled his thumb out of his mouth long enough to greet the boys in the group. Briefly acknowledging him, they formed a semi-circle to prevent him from entering their play. Frustrated, he quickly stepped around them and kicked their structure over. They yelled for help, and Leticia from her cutting station loudly reprimanded him, telling him to find someplace else to go. Harold, just inside from getting the yard ready, called to him, "Come help me put the bikes out, Leo." Leo excitedly went over to him and grabbed him by the hand as they went outside. Several of the other children wanted to go put bikes out too, but Stacey became annoyed and announced it was clean-up time.

Although Marsha's seeming focus is on Leo, she is primarily interested in the adults' ability to respond to him. She is equally interested in the providers' interactions with all of the children. The consultant takes these snippets of information and begins to formulate ideas about the adults' functioning and abilities. What stops Leticia from responding to Leo's physical and emotional bids for connection? How does Harold respond so easily? The consultant is also looking for moments for future intervention and assessing the adults' skill level in responding.

Because we are currently considering the consultant's efforts to get to know the program and its individuals, Leo's behavior does not hold center stage. Of course, Marsha is aware of Leo's experience, but her observation is designed to cull information about the program as a whole. If and when Leo becomes the focus of a case consultation, Marsha will use the incidents in which he seeks physical connection and unsuccessfully tries to enter his peers' play to highlight his dependence on the staff and to engender empathy for his experience. Marsha will help Stacey and Leticia, who can't step far enough back to observe him objectively, to see his neediness and his difficulty expressing it. She will also connect this to his family relationships, revealing a more complex picture to which Leticia, Stacy, and Harold may have a greater chance of relating. The consultant stores her ideas about Leo. Her lens of consideration expands to take in all she can about the program's philosophy and practice and the providers' styles and skills with all children.

The children had difficulty settling for circle time. Stacey looked up sheepishly and said with a shrug, "The beginning of the year." Marsha nodded in acknowledgment, attempting to be reassuring, but Stacey remained nervous. Leticia seemed particularly harsh with the children as she scolded them to sit down, "Criss-cross, apple-sauce." Marsha had heard that expression before but never knew what it was supposed to mean. Apparently, neither did the children. Leticia repeated herself again and again. Finally, most of the children were ready. Leo took a place in the circle and the children moved away from him. "Keep your hands to yourself," Leticia scolded him. She was standing outside the circle policing, but Leo hadn't actually touched anyone.

Stacey began circle time and really lit up. Marsha enjoyed watching her. The children participated gleefully as they introduced themselves and sang songs. Even Leo seemed to enjoy this, but Leticia scolded him repeatedly for squirming: he always wanted to sit closer to his peers. At the 20-minute mark, many of the children had become distracted. Leticia barked instructions from across the room, but by this point few of the children complied. (Harold and she were setting up tables for small group activities.) Stacey's enthusiastic and animated rendition of a story she was reading captivated the group a bit longer. By 45 minutes, Stacey's skills, however formidable, were no match for the 3- and 4-year-olds' attention spans—the children were moving, getting scolded, and losing outside time fast. Exasperated, Stacey ended the group abruptly. The children were assigned to three groups and clustered around an equal number of tables for a structured activity time.

In the move to small groups, Leo got lost again. He wandered around the room while Leticia lectured him on the importance of listening. Although what she said made sense, she seemed to say it more for appearances—Leo had not taken in one word. As he passed by Harold, Harold gently scooped him into his group. The project didn't seem that well planned, but Harold had effectively engaged his group of boys, most of whom had just been in trouble. Group assignment had seemed arbitrary at the time, but over the course of a few visits, the consultant realized that Stacey chose groups to showcase her skills. Her easy-to-engage group was producing some interesting artwork with the materials she had clearly invested energy preparing. Leticia had spent time during free play cutting out shapes; now she was firmly directing each child to produce uniform pictures that she would later hang up proudly. Noticing the consultant's eyes on Leticia, Stacey raised her eyebrows dramatically so that Marsha could see her disdain.

Marsha needed a moment outside the class to consider what she had seen so far. Preparing the class for her leave-taking, Marsha exited. Harold entered the staff room while Marsha was jotting down notes. They greeted each other. Marsha commented on the special connection he seemed to have with many of the kids. She wondered how he had gotten so good with kids. Harold smiled but stayed quiet. For a few moments they sat together in silence. Because it was Friday, Marsha asked if he was looking forward to the weekend. Harold brightened. His preschool-age grandson was going to be visiting this weekend. Harold puffed with pride as he talked about his grandson and how he helped his son and daughter-in-law with understanding their child's development. Marsha wondered about how he let them know. Initially, his daughter-in-law had lived with them but left because she thought Harold and his wife were too critical. "I've been a lot more careful lately. I might say something to my son, but I'm careful not to criticize. He's our only grandson, and my wife has warned me." They laughed, and Marsha commented on the complexity of family life. Harold continued, "Now, I just put out things that I think he'll like. Then they ask questions." Marsha offered, "I imagine that's easier for all of you. Sounds like your son and daughter-in-law are interested in your ideas when they are the ones asking for your expertise. I think that's true for most of us, don't you?"

Harold relaxed significantly and began to tell her that he actually never planned on working with kids and as a new parent he had no experience. He had worked at a number of maintenance jobs for years, but then he lost his job. A friend suggested that there was an opening at this program. He had expected a janitorial position, but it turned out they needed an assistant teacher. At the time, Harold said there were all African-American children and it was good to have an African-American male role model. Marsha agreed that child care benefited from having both. He admitted that he had been a troubled kid who had needed a stronger male presence. Marsha responded that he had a lot of experience but noted that he had remained so quiet at the meeting. "As long as I've worked with children, I've been here. Some of the kids I've worked with are now parents here. Since I started I've seen several directors and just as many head teachers come and go. I've learned it's best to keep quiet and hang back. I just watch and let other people do the deciding." "Laying low seems to have served a purpose? It's just that you seem to have so much knowledge and experience, I wouldn't want me or your coworkers to miss out on what you have to offer. If it's okay, I may ask you in the meetings what you think. But, if you don't want to answer just let me know. Will that work for you?" Harold acquiesced and they parted. Marsha didn't realize at this meeting, but their most important conversations were going to occur casually, right in this room.

Some think of consultation as a weekly meeting, some observations, and expert advice. However, consultation can occur in every interaction. Harold may not be responsive in meetings, but he does have a unique perspective as an African-American male, a former inexperienced parent, and a child who had difficulties. But drawing on this expertise can be challenging, especially when offering ideas has been seen as criticism, as Harold has described. Marsha must create a safe space for him to voice his opinions. For the moment, the place may exist only in private conversations. Stacey, who values her formal education, may not be able to appreciate Harold's knowledge, which is based on intuition and life experience. However, Marsha does not ignore his reluctance to participate. She comments on his valuable contribution and follows with direct questions about his silence in the meeting. She respects this silence by assuring him that he has the final decision about how to participate but seeks permission to ask for his contribution. By solidifying this arrangement, Marsha encourages an expansion of his involvement that will hopefully build his confidence. In turn, and by her example, Harold's participation may lead to greater respect from his colleagues and requests for his input. Eventually, the consultant seeks to expand the channels of communication among all of the staff.

> On her way back to the classroom, Marsha passed Leticia going to the break room for another cup of coffee. Marsha was surprised she noticed but that had to be at least the fourth cup of coffee. Leticia left the room often.

Weaving together these thin threads of experience, the consultant begins to construct a portrait of each staff member. Leticia's frequent forays to the lounge, her robotic cutting of paper towels, and her distant but critical supervision of children outline a pessimistic picture. As Marsha fills in this picture, she will want to understand the reasons for Leticia's distance. She will look for clues that answer her questions. Is Leticia's life personally overwhelming? Does she like children? Does she enjoy her job and coworkers? How does she understand the children and her role with them? Does she dismiss others as unimportant because she feels similarly discounted? As Marsha gets to know Leticia better, she may ask some of these questions directly—always expressing the wish to understand Leticia more fully.

> Back in the classroom, the children were just going down for a nap. Marsha watched Leo struggle on his cot. He didn't seem ready to settle in to sleep. The more he struggled the more Stacey raised her voice. Each seemed to antagonize the other. Neither could calm down. Marsha strained to contain herself too, but finally picking up a book, she went over to Leo and asked him if he wanted her to read to him. She whispered the story to him as he leaned against her. Burrowing into her body, he took her arm and wrapped himself in it. Eventually, Leo lay down and she patted him until he fell asleep.

> In supervision, Marsha confessed how proud she was for helping and for showing how easily this could be done. "You learned a lot about what Leo needs. I wonder what the teachers made of your involvement?" asked her supervisor. Immediately, Marsha realized that she had overstepped her bounds in her efforts to be responsive. Marsha had watched helplessly as

Leo struggled in an environment that wasn't well-suited for him. What Marsha knew best was how to help children directly—how could she resist? With her supervisor's guidance, Marsha explored her motivation further. She recognized that she also wanted to prove herself an expert in this program brimming with experienced early childhood professionals. The combination of powerlessness and the desire to show competence had been overwhelming. The supervisor asked how, in retrospect, Marsha would have wished to behave. The supervisor reassured Marsha that there would be opportunity to acknowledge and correct her missteps as she would be returning week after week to consult.

Now Marsha had to go back. A meeting had been scheduled for the following week, after she had observed the classroom twice. She shared some of her thoughts with Patricia, and they worked together on the agenda for the meeting. Patricia preferred that Marsha lead the meeting. Again, the participants straggled into the meeting. Patricia had to track down Stacey. Although he seemed engaged, Harold still sat outside the group. Sitting inside the circle, Stacey removed herself by working on her curriculum planning. Marsha wondered how it had been having her observe and got a curt "fine" from all. Leticia hoped that Marsha would intervene with Leo more. "That's funny," Marsha, relieved to have the opening, observed, "I've been thinking a lot about having hopped in to help when none of you had asked me to. I now have a sense of Leo, but at the same time, I missed the more important part. I didn't get to see what you, who know him so well, would have done. Besides, a helpful moment counts for very little when what we need to do is understand enough of what contributes to a child's distress so that you feel better equipped to manage the daily dilemma. I could see how challenging he is and what I did may have only worked because I'm new." Tuning in, Stacey said, "That's true. He woke up soon after you left and was twice as much trouble." "So it wasn't helpful" Marsha asked nondefensively. Stacey responded, "No, what you did worked, but we don't have time to give each child that kind of attention." Marsha agreed. Knowing that it was premature, she resisted the desire to point out that only a few children seemed to need that kind of attention. Marsha also noted how frustrating her intervention must have seemed because it gave Stacey the idea that Marsha didn't understand how challenging her job with Leo was. Stacey nodded acceptance.

Despite a consultant's best efforts, her involvement in a center may initially feel intrusive. Staff meetings are an extra burden until their worth seems evident. Classroom observations can feel exposing and raise undue anxiety until the information gathered from them can be used to bring relief. Consequently, additional uninvited involvement of the consultant, like Marsha's intervention with Leo, can be unsettling and unintentionally communicate criticism. Furthermore, stepping in can also alter perceptions and expectations for the consultant's role. For example, Leticia's wondering if she will "work on the floor" reveals her own wish to have the burdens of the classroom eased but also the shifting perception of Marsha's possible contributions.

Marsha observes the struggle and asks about it directly. With her questioning, she offers possible interpretations of her misstep, alerting Stacey and the others that she can acknowledge her mistakes and tolerate the staff's views. The consultant hopes that her openness models her faith in the process and the collaborative nature of consultation. She will consider the providers' input and tailor her actions accordingly. This does not mean that the consultant indiscriminately adapts her stance just because a new way of working is requested. She has neither offered nor plans to directly intervene with children. However, she does consider those requests and wonders about the underlying hopes that they contain.

As her supervisor had advised, Marsha abandoned her idea to broach the lengthy circle time, the disorganized naptime, and the challenges of the small groups. Instead she invited the staff to help her understand their frustrations. Everyone, including Harold, chimed in to complain about Leo at circle time, Leo at naptime, and Leo in small groups. Harold was the only one to temper his complaints with attempts to understand Leo's experience of home and preschool. By noting his success with Leo, Marsha inadvertently encouraged Harold to share that he too was a kid who had trouble in school and he just wanted to make it easier for Leo. Stacey revealed her surprise at Harold's personal revelation because he rarely spoke about his experiences. Although Marsha appreciated their frustration and their thoughtfulness, she recognizes that they have not received permission from Leo's mother to discuss him in as much depth as the staff would like. She attempts to broaden the discussion. Although Leo demonstrated distress most clearly, several children struggled with the extended circle time and unclear transitions. Marsha generalizes to all the children: "I know Leo shows his distress in big ways, but do you ever notice other children having difficulty staying in circle time? Stacey you are really masterful at maintaining the children's interest, but you seemed dismayed when children started to stray at the end. It must be frustrating to have it fizzle out when you clearly put a lot of thought into how circle time goes. I can imagine resenting the children who can't show their appreciation of your thoughtful plan. Tell me about your ideas and the purpose of circle time. Maybe we could think of ways to reach those goals so that both you and the children felt satisfied." After she gives Stacey a chance to respond, she turns to the other staff members and elicits their ideas. Stacey explains that she needs to occupy the children while Harold and Leticia set up activities. Marsha wondered if Leticia and Harold could take up some of the burden. Harold unexpectedly offered to include some of the children in setting up, especially those who got antsy early. Marsha thought that this was a brilliant solution because it would relieve the tension in circle time and provide a secondary benefit—it would give Leo and others like him the attention they need with the person most equipped to help. By framing the plan as relief for Stacey, Marsha made it possible for Stacey to accept the suggestion and the assistance. On her way out, Stacey admitted, "That was helpful."

Throughout her meetings with the staff and her observations, Marsha has seemingly focused on Leo. As we have suggested, however, her scope is much greater. She will address Leo's challenges specifically, but she also uses him as a conduit to better understand the staff. Reciprocally, this new-found comprehension will help her to better serve the staff in their attempts to improve the program and Leo's functioning.

Although Harold's designation as Leo's primary caregiver in the classroom relieves Stacey and Leticia from shifting their stance in the classroom and may be an additional burden for Harold, the new status as the go-to-guy may offset these drawbacks. Marsha will need to attend to how Harold interprets any expansion in his role and responsibilities as the year proceeds. For the moment, this may be the most expedient and effective way to address Leo's needs and provide needed staff relief, but the consultant will also need to find ways to involve the women.

Leo offered a challenge to the teaching staff, which for the most part they resented. Marsha's willingness to acknowledge, to label, and to accept their resentment allowed them to consider more fully not only Leo's but other children's experience. Her acceptance along with her inquisitiveness allowed them to find their own path of understanding. Their own solution is ultimately more satisfying than any Marsha could have offered. Furthermore, their investment in the proposed adaptations will be greater than had Marsha recommended them. Of course, the solutions are consistent with Marsha's goals of enhancing the program, and she did guide them there through wondering with them, labeling the subjective experience of all the participants, and being attentive to her own role and contributions and to others' perceptions of her.

Summary

The process of "getting to know" can be difficult to balance for a consultant who needs to be both a part of the relationships in the program and yet watch herself and the others from outside. Maintaining equilibrium among the providers' various expectations for the consultant and her work, the individual personalities, and the program's challenges can be daunting because they are constantly shifting as the consultant and the providers come to know each other. Through the consultant's relationships with the program and each of its members and her observations of the others' relationships with the children and with each other, the consultant comes to understand a program. In addition to her observations, she employs direct questions and develops hypotheses that she continues to test as she gathers more information. During this stage, she is coming to understand the subjective experiences of the adults and children so that she might help them to communicate more effectively. To develop that knowledge, the consultant needs to familiarize herself with the general expectations and perceptions of her and each other, the program's philosophy of care, the organizational structure, and the individuals' roles and relationships. As in every stage of the consultation, relationships are both the focus as well as the method of the consultative efforts.

Chapter 4

Addressing Process
Through Content

In previous chapters, we have seen how a child-care mental health consultant set the stance, entered a child-care program, established the best vantage point from which to view the proceedings, and began to explore how to stand there. Now we delve further into the process of consultation. How does a consultant move within the confines of a child-care program's rules, system, and philosophy to create change when a drive to maintain the status quo is a defining characteristic of all institutions? We revisit some of the principles outlined in earlier chapters and apply them to particular child-care situations. Specifically, we explore applications of the concept of "wondering, not knowing." We again reference subjective experience, looking at how voicing each participant's perspective can build empathy among caregivers and break down resistance to change. First, we examine all the levels of influence on child-care providers' practices.

Although providers generally find it easier to embrace consultation that is directed at an individual child, discussion of program practices that affect all children is the only way to change a system. Program consultation necessarily addresses a range of areas, including, among others, interstaff communication, curriculum development, organizational philosophy, and expectations for children. Over time, a consultant might talk with a director about supervising the staff, engaging parents in the program, and appropriately gearing classroom practices to the children's skills and abilities, as well as administrative issues.

Because a number of well-researched and theoretically sound early childhood education texts exist (Bredekamp & Copple, 1997; Klugman & Smilansky, 1991; Lally, Griffin, Fenichel, Segal, Szanton, & Weissbourd, 1995; Seefeldt, 1999), we will not try to describe or analyze here the range of child-care programs' philosophies, environmental conditions, and configurations of staff. Instead, we offer a consultative approach that considers and addresses myriad aspects of early childhood education and finds ways to circumvent impediments to quality care. Our approach to consultation is designed to help child-care providers develop and fulfill their own ideals of quality care—which is not to dismiss the consultant's values. The types and level of intervention necessary to change a child-care program's system vary. Some programs need help to develop a cohesive vision of care. Many programs already have a well-developed philosophy but haven't been able to reach their goals. Through inquiry and exploration, the consultant helps to find out why. The process of program consultation helps child-care staff to identify obstacles to implementing best practices and, when things go well, to surmount them.

We believe that the quality of relationships between all members of a child-care community predicts, in large measure, the overall quality of care. However, most child-care professionals lack a mental health perspective on human behavior, interaction, and systemic functioning that would help them strengthen relationships and thereby improve quality. Mental health professionals are trained to decipher and address relationships. Therefore, the dynamic process of consultation offers child-care providers an additional path to high-quality care for all children in their program. To understand where opportunities for change in a child-care program exist, we must first consider the levels of influence on child-care practice.

Considering Levels of Influence

Improving the quality of relationships within a child-care community, especially the child–provider relationship, is the ultimate aim of consultation. However, this relationship does not occur in a vacuum. It cannot be meaningfully considered separate from the forces that shape its unfolding. The sheer number of children in child-care programs and the increasing number of hours they spend there each day and each week means that child-care programs are expected to assume responsibility for more and more caregiving functions. The factors contributing to child care's expanded role can also strain the system. Outlining the particular pressures (both real and perceived) in specific child-care programs becomes crucial to understanding the individuals involved, the types and intensity of the stresses that they are experiencing, and the resulting decisions that they make about the children in their care. We will start by describing relatively distant spheres of influence, such as social forces and government policies, and circle in until we approach the child-care provider's family life and relationships with her coworkers. Each influence has a bearing on how—and how well—a program functions. All are considered in consultation.

Social and Political Forces

Currently, American society as a whole massively undervalues out-of-home child care. The repercussions of this underappreciation reverberate through the child-care system and are reflected in providers' self-perceptions as well as their paychecks. Research (Cost, Quality and Outcomes Study Team, 1995; Whitebrook, Howes, & Phillips, 1988, 1989) on quality underscores the systemic implications of an undercompensated child-care workforce. Among adult work variables in child care, the level of staff wages is the most significant predictor of quality (Cost, Quality and Outcome Study Team, 1995). Other leading indicators of quality include adult–child ratio, group size, caregiver continuity, and caregiver training. When the ratio of children to caregivers and the number of children in a group size swell to cover the cost, quality of care deteriorates. High staff turnover because of low pay further degrades the system.

Monetary devaluing is symbolic of broader disregard for child care. Caring for children is not seen as a skilled profession that requires expertise. As a consequence, child-care staff often enter the field with inadequate training and work for low wages throughout their careers. Child-care staff who stay in programs may do so out of desperation, but most stay out of dedication. However, providers can eventually internalize the societal message of devaluation. Their sense of self-efficacy and professional esteem suffer if caregivers lack day-to-day support and opportunities for professional development. By extension, child-care staff find it difficult to respect their coworkers in an undervalued endeavor. In sum, the personal sacrifices of child-care providers subsidize child care in the United States. American society as a whole seems to find this situation acceptable. We believe, however, that ignoring the real costs of child care (and who pays them) serves no one well, especially children. In spite of these significant social pressures, most providers comport themselves with dignity. They convey to children a sense that the relationships they create together are valuable. Caregivers' ability to build and sustain meaningful relationships in conditions of such adversity is a personal achievement, a professional accomplishment, and an act with political and social implications.

Local, State, and Federal Guidelines

With the changes in welfare reform and the increases in the number of working parents, the need for government funding to provide child care for the working poor has increased. With this funding come new rules and regulations for child care. Child-care programs interpret these rules idiosyncratically as they implement them. For example, in subsidized child care each child is required to have a file; assessments and written observations are to be made regularly. How these are enacted varies from program to program. Other centers are required to report data about the children and their families—some programs will have a designated person with allotted time to accomplish these tasks, but others will place these obligations on the child-care providers without additional time or compensation. Different communities vary in the resources offered and the regulations imposed.

As with any guideline, the underlying reasons for its existence may be forgotten in strict adherence to the letter of the law. Sometimes requirements (or their interpretations) don't reflect the needs of the children or even consider their development. Sometimes government pressures are passed on unknowingly. With increased testing and standards for school-age children and the resulting increase in expectations for teachers, the pressure on child-care providers has inadvertently been increased without being identified, depending on the school district and school–child-care relationship. Because literacy and school readiness can be narrowly interpreted as the acquisition of rote academic skills, kindergarten teachers often expect that children will arrive with the ability to identify and write all their letters, read a few words, and count. Although this may be developmentally beyond many children and certainly for those in at-risk communities, child-care providers who fail to reach these milestones with their children are considered inept. These criticisms often result in "academically" driven program practices that unintentionally stress children—especially when the knowledge of child development is lacking and the self-efficacy of teachers is low. In the teaching profession, as the age of a teacher's children decreases, so does her value. Child-care providers suffer under this system and sometimes institute practices to bolster their self-esteem at the expense of children. Some may institute overly long circle times to rehearse letters and numbers in order to address these perceived areas of inadequacy. Often, this practice results in less success with children and increased frustration for both provider and child.

At other times, minimum requirements can be interpreted as satisfactory or even replace better practices. For instance, the attempt to protect children from abductors and child-care programs' liability produced the sign-in sheet. In some programs, parents and teachers revert to the sign-in sheet as a form of communication. The morning greeting is forgotten, even though it would actually serve as a better protector of a child and help to facilitate transition and greater consistency between home and school.

Government expectations come through funding requirements, incentives, and licensing requirements. The intentions are most always positive ones but sometimes not reflective of the real demands of child care or typical child development. The pressure to respond to these requirements can result in misguided approaches that seem inexplicable unless one understands the expectations that generated them.

Bureaucracy

Of course, a program's pressures can also be internal. These program policy issues, site-specific constraints, and funding-related demands have consequences for the provider–child relationship and on consultation.

A few classrooms surrounding a small outside play space might require juggling and limiting outside time for each, meeting no one's needs for movement and mobility. Another school, with limited funds and bare-bones staff, has everyone outside for longer than anyone can tolerate in order to stretch staffing and meet ratio requirements. Naptime is the ubiquitous bureaucratic imperative that solves the staffing challenge of breaks and shift changes.

These challenges will also impede the consultation. An understaffed, underfunded program may not be able to set aside time for staff to meet. Identifying these bureaucratic hurdles will help in distinguishing them from resistance to the consultant or to her interventions. Of course, these roadblocks sometimes serve the staff for they offer tangible reasons for resisting change. In our experience, 50% of the programs that we entered had no times to meet. Only after programs came to see the consultant and talking to one another as useful did they begin institutionalizing time for staff meetings. Wondering about a program's bureaucracy will foster a sense of empathy for the staff's predicaments and also serve to differentiate actual programmatic obstacles from historically held habits.

Community

At the center of any vibrant community with a desire to grow and to improve lie children as the impetus for change. Conversely, the community's struggles and limitations will shape the child-care program and its children. Is the neighborhood a safe one? Does it have playgrounds? If so, are they littered with hypodermic needles or are they pristine? What is the level of violence? Decisions about the children's engagement with the surrounding environment will be based on the answers. For instance, walks to explore may be too treacherous. How do the children arrive at the center—by car, by public transportation, or by foot? The answer will affect everything from the occasional field trip to the daily pick-up and drop-off time to the child's morning disposition and readiness to leave. It will influence the school's hours of opening and rules around lateness. The community's general economic status and access to resources will echo in the child-care setting. In turn, the child-care center can serve as a haven or replicate the overwhelming aspects of the surrounding environment and, with luck, can offer a meeting place for community advocacy, parent support, and respite.

A child-care center's functioning is intimately linked with that of the community. We have listed only a few of the multitude of environmental influences on a program. Consultation requires detective work to observe and ferret out the community's functioning and to find the connections to the child-care center's decisions, treatment of children, and general health. Drawing those connections in a group effort with caregivers may be the first opportunity that they have had to consider the impact on the children or even themselves. However, the receptivity of providers will depend on their place in the community—closely linked by membership to the outside or unaware of the community at-large. Members of a staff will fall everywhere along that spectrum, and their willingness to consider these environmental influences will depend on their acceptance of their place in the community and their tolerance for feelings of powerlessness, pain, and guilt.

Parents' Contributions

Individually, parents will act out aspects of the community in their relationships with the child-care provider. Can they be engaged and supportive or are they overpowered by their experiences with little left to engage their child's caregivers let alone their children? One private suburban child care has parents lined up overnight, sleeping in their cars, on the evening prior to the first day of enrollment while another subsidized program cannot predict their population's stability as they serve primarily homeless families. The first takes a tremendous amount of parents' fortitude and financial resources, reflected in the center's cost and functioning, while the latter's financial health and daily routine depend on parents' ability to plan and persevere in the face of daily upheaval and limited personal control. The expectations for parent contribution will affect the parent culture. Parents in the program will also affect each other's contributions, encouraging or discouraging participation and support of the program. In turn, the parents' functioning can be fostered or hindered by the child-care center's interpretation of the parents' lack of, or wealth of, participation. Does the program invite parent participation or shun it? The level of parent inclusion and welcome will shape not only parents' support of the program and their children but their receptivity to consultation. If parents trust and feel a part of the child-care community, the consultant likely benefits from this established atmosphere of inclusion. Being introduced as another member of a supportive network at a program's beginning-of-the-year open house sets a significantly different tone than having to eke out every introduction to parents who may be suspicious of an outsider.

Providers' Personal Experience

The parents of children are not the only family members participating in the child-care setting. The staff members have their own social circumstances that inform their practices and classroom choices. Family schedules and responsibilities will influence a teacher's engagement, willingness, and ability to be flexible around schedule. Staying late to accommodate a parent's work hours so that an essential meeting can occur may simply be impossible—no matter the teacher's wish to be accommodating. In addition, current relationships with their own families, both positive and negative, will enter the program through ideas about children, general stress level, and emotional availability, among others. A mother who must leave her infant to care for someone else's may not be able to respond to the cries of her charges because of the emotional conflict it causes. Knowing these important dimensions of a provider's personal life can keep a consultant from becoming disillusioned or, alternately, demanding the impossible. The consultant's capacity to respond empathically expands as she comprehends the provider's reality; in turn, the consultant's efficacy increases.

Ghosts in the Nursery School

Providers' ideas about child rearing and their subsequent behavior with children are influenced not only by their current circumstances and training but also by their own early experiences. Often a provider's internally held beliefs, created by the ways in which she was raised by her family and through her culture and by her accumulation of experiences in the world, exert more power than years of training. Being human, providers bring all of who they are and how they have been treated to their professional relationships. Various views of child rearing and development, characteristic styles of relating, flexible or fixed expectations of others, and emotional strengths and vulnerabilities will be played out in relationships on the child-care stage. The idea that complex intrapsychic phenomena are carried into work relationships is not surprising, nor is it an assumed liability, but it must be considered, especially when these phenomena interfere with the creation of positive and, for children, essentially enhancing relationships.

All parents can relate to the broken promise, "I will never say what my parents said to me to my children." However, in moments of stress, one unintentionally relies on the ingrained, even when it has been hurtful. The same is perhaps more true for the child-care provider who is taxed by the needs of many children. Sometimes despite years of education, a child-care provider will fall back on the familiar. On a particularly hard day, one teacher raises her voice to scare the children into submission despite her belief that clear and consistent reminders will be more effective in the long run. The pressures of the moment can overwhelm the best intentions.

Unconscious re-enactment of past experience can further complicate the child-care setting. Even when someone can intellectually acknowledge a better scenario, an unconscious push to repeat or to master the past intercedes. For instance, a teacher who embraced the school's philosophy of child-directed free play grew up in a home with rigid rules and an extremely strict hierarchy with great emphasis on respect for adults. Even though she could speak eloquently about (and believed in) children's need for exploration, independence, and self-expression, she squelched their attempts by directing play, demanding adherence to rules, and forbidding negotiation. To her colleagues and the consultant, her words and actions were inconsistent, but she did not see the contradiction. She interpreted her ideas through the lens of her childhood experience.

Occasionally, a teacher's lens (created through accumulated past experience) can cause more serious interference. Another teacher was blind to the signs of abuse in children, in one instance unwittingly concealing evidence of abuse from other teachers and unintentionally allying with the injury-inflicting parent. Despite extensive training, several warnings, and her own insistence that she wanted to intercede, the teacher's distortions kept her from seeing the severity of the situation. Through consultation, she revealed her own experience of abuse, one she had previously discounted. Acknowledging the serious maltreatment of her charge meant accepting the horrors of her own history and allowing for the anger and pain that came with remembering. Reporting the abuse also opened the possibility of the child's removal from her home. Although the teacher's own mistreatment was severe and most likely would have warranted separation, she was terrified, even retrospectively, of the idea that she could have been taken from her mother by whom she desperately wanted to be loved rather than shunned. Removal would have confirmed her worst fears and dashed her greatest hope—connection with her mother—then and now. Consultants have to be aware of these interfering intrapsychic influences and carefully construct pathways to awareness.

In an attempt to describe the pitfalls of the ghosts in the nursery, we do not want to discount the positive affects of early childhood experiences. Although we notice the consequences of negative early childhood experiences on child-care practices more often, positive early childhood experiences contribute just as much if not more to the success of child care. Responding intuitively and sensitively to the needs of children is an art often gained through the experience of feeling cared for and loved. Although training, self-awareness, and intention may prepare caregivers for caring for young children, "being in tune" with a child is an invaluable skill that is most often felt rather than learned.

Culture

Every aspect of human existence is woven with and altered by culture. To some degree, culture governs the ways in which each person (a) thinks, feels, and expresses emotion; (b) experiences and organizes time and space; and (c) perceives and solves problems. Although cultural influences in child care cannot be neatly parsed from personal histories or characteristic modes of interacting, its importance warrants separate consideration.

Appreciation of culture in child care is often limited to concrete manifestations such as food preferences and holiday celebrations. Cultural variations and experiences of child-rearing practices, affective expression, language, and learning more deeply impact relationships in child care but are less often considered. Although culture is at play in every interaction in child care, it often comes to light only in terms of discord as alternate expressions rub up against each other.

Anticipating and honoring differences, a consultant creates an atmosphere in which disagreement, when it arises, can be openly explored. The consultant's ability to do so is predicated on her awareness of her own cultural beliefs and biases. She attends to differences in language, ethnicity, religion, and immigration history. In addition, the culture of child care is distinct and powerful. In many respects and for many reasons, child care mimics the dominant Northern European culture. Verbal communication, routines prescribed by a linear timeframe, and autonomy are encouraged. These beliefs have ordained a set of "developmentally appropriate" practices that may be more reflective of the majority culture's beliefs and attitudes than actual child development. Ascribing greater or lesser importance to this value system is not the issue, but consultants can carry an awareness of these structurally sanctioned views and appraise their fit with the providers and families embedded in the system.

Staff Relationships

Finally, all these components converge on an essential relationship in the care of young children—the ones between the caregivers. The ways in which staff members interact will change the course of each of their days and ultimately shape their contact with children. Caregivers' zeal for the day depends on how they anticipate their work—with dread or with eagerness. Each of the previous levels of influence contributes, but it is the ongoing relationships with coworkers and with the children and their families that sustain enthusiasm for the work. Consultation often begins with and returns to consider the influence of staff relationships on the quality of care. Along the way the consultant integrates the other influencing factors in her interpretations and decision making. This final and tightest sphere in child care, however, always remains in focus.

Staff relations are affected by two sets of circumstances: (a) the interface of the individuals' varied, longstanding values and beliefs and (b) the moment-to-moment emotional shifts of those who are intertwined for many hours each day in a highly interpersonal endeavor. As discussed earlier, providers bring their unique visions, derived from equally idiosyncratic cultural and personal pasts and present experiences, to their relationships with each other. Their interpretations of the behavior of children and each other are largely based on these views. Because different caregivers' experiences, and thus their values and beliefs, vary, there are potential misunderstandings. These are magnified by child care's requirement of working particularly closely and cooperatively.

In addition, the intimacy of caring for young children evokes a wide range of intense feelings. These emotions engage defenses that extend from rigidly avoiding feelings to endlessly and profusely exuding affect. Because child care is an intensely personal and intimate endeavor, caregivers must manage these feelings for themselves and with each other. Providers' affective states shift in response to children; such a shift may ripple among the caregivers. For instance, in a primary caregiving arrangement for infants, a crying baby evokes two different responses from the two caregivers working cooperatively to care for a total of six infants. One provider's experience of early deprivation leads her to believe that quickly dispatched comfort spoils children so she avoids the distress. The other provider, who does not have primary responsibility for this infant, finds the infant's bids impossible to ignore. Finally, agitated and outraged, she picks up the infant, violating both her agreement with her coworker and her coworker's values. Tensions rise between the two due to their emotional responses, which inform and are informed by their values and beliefs.

Revisiting Stance

We have briefly introduced the multiple influences affecting daily child-care experience—everything from bureaucratic pressures to intrapsychic forces and from intimate interpersonal exchanges to overall community functioning. To uncover all of these areas immediately would be daunting. Instead, they are areas for consideration and may reveal themselves with time. Nevertheless, the consultant must be aware of these contributing factors to identify them as they arise. More importantly, how does one come to know and incorporate what one is learning in the consultative process? Process is the operative word. Let's begin there.

The title of this chapter—*Addressing Process Through Content*—reverses most approaches to process. Process usually moves toward achievement or goals, but here process is the goal. Because the measurement of achievement in consultation (at least as we conceptualize it) is the quality and intensity of relationships, especially the child–provider relationship, process is essential for observing, identifying, and addressing those relationship challenges. Process refers to dynamic development, involving many changes in individuals, relationships, and systems. We work within relationships because we believe that change occurs through relationships.

Several process components are important toward building satisfying relationships: (a) identifying the factors influencing behavior—both the children's and the adults'; (b) acknowledging the effect on practices; (c) assessing whether the impact is wished for by providers and is benefiting children; (d) adjusting to enhance mutual respect and understanding among adults; and (e) shifting perspective on a child or program issue. Throughout, involving all the participants in a dialogue about their and others' perceptions reassesses these aspects.

Process involves careful consideration rather than immediate action and assumes understanding before doing. This is often an unfamiliar way of proceeding for many of us, including child-care professionals. It may feel, at least at first, tedious and trying. Consultants as well as providers can feel adrift in a sea of inaction; consequently, finding a focus for attention lessens anxiety. Tethering the somewhat amorphous notion of process to a mutually identified and specific content area gives form and meaning to consultation conversations. Content can come in the form of sorting out a staffing snafu, planning program practices, or discussing a child or parent whose behavior is perplexing.

We have already explored the components of stance, but it may be helpful to delve further into those most applicable to this transformation of content to process. Central to all our work is the concept of wondering, not knowing. Almost every interaction begins here: How did you make that decision? What do you think will happen? How do you understand it?

Wondering, Not Knowing

Stopping to wonder about a crisis can be frustrating, when what might feel most comforting is having an answer. Both consultants and providers can become impatient with "not knowing." Child care can exhaust the most energetic adults, making the daily problem dire. Rarely are good decisions made from this vantage point, yet stopping to think in these moments appears inefficient. Balancing these forces becomes the consultant's trial.

The consultant must convey two ideas: (a) Understanding precedes effective action, and (b) understanding will not necessarily make more work. Both ideas are hard to sell. In an already difficult job, providers attempt to protect themselves from added effort. They fear that understanding a child better may increase feelings of responsibility and take special handling. Shifting a routine for one child feels like an exceptional effort and makes providers resistant to discussion. Change, no matter how minor, is rarely embraced easily. Providers often hope children will adapt with little alteration in adult action. We know that a subtle shift in how a child is seen will increase patience and be mirrored in the child–adult dynamic. In the pulls of this dynamic, rarely does knowing more seem possible. Additionally, the adults' desire to be understood can compete with the child's. The consultant attempts both. Her efforts to wonder about the adults' experiences model and encourage their wondering.

The benefits of pondering reasons for behavior, feelings, or situations are not immediately apparent. However, randomly embarking on responses for the sake of doing something actually prolongs the process because the target is undefined and elusive. Intervention informed by understanding may initially take time but is ultimately more efficient and beneficial.

Exploration embarked upon through "wondering" questions leads to a fuller understanding of a programmatic problem or a conundrum with a child. By asking rather than assuming, the consultant conveys that all behavior has meaning. By inquiring about the meaning or reason for an individual's reactions, the consultant learns the provider's intentions. The provider is asked to consider and become aware, often for the first time, of the reasons for or influences upon behavior. Only through this process can one hope to shift, disabuse, or expand on another's ideas.

Understanding Others' Subjective Experience

In the process of wondering, not knowing, we are always trying to get to another tenet—understanding the subjective experiences of others. The consultant helps the people she works with to find their voice. She also gives voice to the people who are not present—usually the children, but sometimes parents and other teachers. In that process, she navigates between these different voices trying to find common ground.

Sometimes direct communication between individuals is not immediately possible even when the consultant assists by translating for the participants. Fears of conflict, interpersonal difficulties, and a lack of empathy may hinder direct expression. Until they are able to communicate directly, the consultant fosters the possibility. First, her belief in and expressed hope for the possibility of shared experience introduces the idea, perhaps for the first time. The consultant's offer of a listening ear may eventually increase the safety and allow for practice before sharing with the group. Also, the experience may make providers more emotionally available to their peers and to the children in their care.

Although the consultant always encourages direct communication, she respects and understands providers' reluctance to speak openly with each other. However, she gently challenges this notion by wondering about expected responses and fears. In some instances, she may speak for others' experience with permission from the participants concerning both for whom and to whom she speaks. Even when she does so, the consultant expresses her wish to have people speak directly with each other and her expectation that some day that will seem possible. She also expects that people have varying levels of tolerance for this sort of dialogue and that intense feelings may arise as previously unvoiced concerns and wishes are uncovered. An example may better illustrate these ideas.

In one center, a supervision crisis arose over absences. The site supervisor, Wendy, who understandably worried about staff–child ratios, demanded regular attendance from her staff. Katrina, a teacher's assistant, had trouble meeting this expectation because of the effects of domestic violence in her home, legitimate illnesses, and her child's difficulties in elementary school, which required regular meetings during school hours. Katrina's challenges were not different from those of the families within the child-care center, which was an asset in these relationships. Parents and children felt immediately comfortable with her because she intimately understood the challenges of the community. She also was intuitively responsive and patient with the most difficult children. Because of Katrina's excessive absences, however, Wendy refused all her requests for time off and was threatening to fire

Katrina. Rather than attempting to negotiate, Katrina regularly called in sick or failed to show up, infuriating Wendy. The consultant found herself in the middle—appreciating Katrina's life challenges and her success as a teacher (which were intricately linked) and Wendy's supervisory duties. Katrina had shared her challenges with the consultant, but her anger and fear of retaliation or rejection prevented her from explaining her absences to Wendy. The consultant could speak to each of the women about the other's general concerns and conundrums but did not yet have permission to specifically share Katrina's problems. With the consultant's help, Katrina could tentatively entertain the notion that sharing her circumstances might be beneficial, but the interactions had become too heated for her to feel safe talking directly to Wendy. The consultant respected and understood Katrina's reluctance as a symptom of her domestic situation and as an accurate assessment of Wendy's current openness to the conversation. With Katrina's permission, the consultant gingerly approached Wendy. It was a delicate balance they needed to explore because, by voicing Katrina's concerns, Wendy felt that the consultant took her side, exacerbating Wendy's feelings of isolation as the site supervisor. Over time, the consultant was able to offer each the other's subjective experience neutrally enough so that neither felt judged. As that became more possible, the consultant arranged for the three of them to meet to discuss these problems, offering a safer environment where each felt understood and feelings were contained. It was a long time before Katrina and Wendy could meet alone to peacefully negotiate a work schedule that was amenable to both, but the consultant's help and expressed (and maintained) hope for direct communication eventually made it possible.

Voicing the subjective experience of each participant is always the consultant's goal, but this may not always be possible. Sometimes, the individual has so successfully submerged feelings in order to protect herself that the consultant's attempts to uncover or give them voice, let alone share them with others, may be too threatening. In other instances, other staff members may not be prepared or emotionally strong enough to tolerate knowledge of their colleagues', or children's internal world. In some programs, the culture may not allow shared feelings. Managers either have expressly forbid these exchanges or have prevented them by eliminating forums for discussion, or the tenor of exchanges may be hostile and feel so uncontrolled that members of the group avoid any unstructured or affect-laden communication. The consultant must consider and respect all these aspects while maintaining the idea that direct communication and shared understanding are possible, necessary, and useful. All the while she is working to create an atmosphere in which mutual exchange is valued.

Mental Health Professionals Suited to Consultation Around Programmatic Issues

Consultation topics range from the specific to the broad and involve individual children and teachers as well as a program's practices and organizational functioning. A consultant is called on to address challenges facing a particular child and find appropriate resources. She may work with the teachers to create more effective circle times or help develop a curriculum for an age group. She might also work on organizational challenges from staffing to training to interstaff relationships. Her work is exhaustive.

No one person could be an expert in all of these areas. Luckily, one need not be. Because the key to consultation lies in the process rather than the specifics, mental health professionals may be best suited for consultation. Although a consultant should have expertise and will have opinions, her primary goal is finding the most amenable outcome for—and as defined by—the consultees.

Mental health professionals are trained to lead process. In addition, they are trained to uncover the motivations and desires of individuals and to identify the impediments to change and the opportunities for intervention. We believe that consultation is not primarily about knowledge but about process—finding the way to knowing. Certainly, other professionals adhere to this tenet and bring this perspective to consultation. Conversely, not all clinicians come with the proper sensitivities or perspective. The issue is one of comfort with ambiguity and an ability to recognize and manage one's own internal responses in order to hold and reflect those of the consultees.

Talking About Difficult Issues and in Awkward Situations

Although we have tried to imbue this rather abstract process of consultation with a measure of reality through the vignettes, it may be helpful to be more specific. Raising the influences on perception and action and exploring individuals' responses and experiences are intimate exchanges that must be broached delicately. Consultants often ask, "How can I say that?" or say, "I can't imagine asking that." Of course, identifying the unspoken meaning in communications and then finding ways to make them apparent is an essential part of consultation. It may be useful, then, to stop here and address these questions. Following are some guidelines with examples from consultation efforts. They are neither exhaustive nor particularly innovative. However, they are necessary.

1. Empathize with the adult's experience. Consultants assume that their primary role is understanding and giving voice to the experience of children. This is essential but not to the exclusion of the adult's experience. Appreciating what providers think and feel and to what they are responding will create openings for the children's experience. Consultants often make the early mistake of giving voice solely to those who have none (i.e., children), but this approach risks alienating the provider. Without ignoring the child's experience, a consultant can also address the provider's.

For instance, as a consultant enters the home of a family child-care provider, she witnesses a toddler being harshly scolded. Putting her hand on the provider's shoulder, she says calmly, "So many children of such varying ages, I imagine it gets really frustrating to entertain all of the children at the same time." Although the verbal focus is brought to the provider's internal experience, two other goals are

119

accomplished in this statement. In addition to her empathy, the consultant has offered a reason for the frustration that is broader than the individual child who is being admonished. Attention to the provider's tone of voice also signals the consultant's expectation that yelling is not the provider's desired way of responding. As the consultant comes to know the provider and her tolerance for discussion, she can layer in the child's reaction. One of our guiding principles has been to voice the subjective experience of all participants in child care, but often the consultant must attend first to the provider. Only as she feels understood can she hear the consultant's interpretation of a child's experience.

2. Find the underlying communication and identify it. Behavior has meaning. This is as true for adults as it is for children. The latter is consistently conveyed, but communicating the former is just as important. This is key to understanding the subjective experience of individuals because rarely do they tell you directly. What, then, is the provider's behavior or response attempting to communicate? Using your own feelings to sort out those of others opens doors to this understanding. In what ways have they shown you how they feel or how they have been treated? What role are you given in their drama, and does it seem to replicate their past experiences? Using your responses can guide you to possible scenarios that you can then test. Then, the consultant must find ways to make the core communications conscious and to express them more directly. In the best circumstances, this act serves two goals: Primarily, the individual feels understood, and secondarily, the consultant demonstrates the benefit of direct communication, raising its value.

Examples elucidate this point. While a consultant observes during a particularly chaotic morning, one staff member takes several children outside, leaving the consultant and a sole provider in the classroom. This teacher immediately exits, calling to the consultant over her shoulder, "Would you watch the children? I need to use the restroom." Without a moment to respond, the consultant is left by herself with 10 children despite the fact that she has told the staff on more than one occasion that she cannot supervise children. Feeling first tricked and then isolated and helpless, the consultant registers her response. Her dismay gives way to greater appreciation for the teacher's dilemma.

The teacher has deftly demonstrated her predicament—too little coverage leaves her with few options to care for herself. Although talking about this problem may have been easier for the consultant, the teacher's action conveys her meaning with greater depth. Now, she and the consultant share the frustration and powerlessness. Rather than asserting the parameters of her position, the consultant might say, "Having so little coverage is really a strain on you. I wonder how you get a break when I'm not here?" Wondering with the teacher brings her attention to the dilemma without asking her to defend her behavior. Again, this takes quick awareness of the consultant's own feelings and ability to translate them to the consultee's message.

A more dramatic example further illustrates the power of underlying communication and the usefulness of identifying it. After anguished consideration, the staff and their consultant decide that their concern about a child's safety warrants reporting. The consultant has encouraged the staff to speak with the child's mother about their decision. Unable to do so, the providers detain the parent as she comes to drop off her child, knowing the consultant will arrive shortly. The unsuspecting parent and the equally unknowing consultant are thrust together in the school's office. As the consultant begins to talk with the parent, the mother dresses her down loudly and long enough for the entire staff to hear the commotion. The consultant feels exposed and manipulated. Her distress is aggravated by the pleasure the staff seems to take in the tumultuous outcome. Although they had not shared their suspicion with the consultant, the staff anticipated this mother's response. That response and the consultant's seeming failure now justify their intense feelings toward the mother. Perhaps, however, a more subtle but important exchange has occurred. The staff may feel that the consultant makes suggestions without fully understanding their experience or their previous attempts. She now has a taste of their fears, frustrations, and perceived short comings.

Although it probably doesn't feel like it in the moment, the situation affords the consultant a valuable opportunity. If she chooses to empathize with the staff's feelings and reframe this sabotage, she will foster greater trust. A good-natured acknowledgement of the fire she passed through with this parent and her feelings of uncertainty and exposure may encourage camaraderie. To further reframe the situation, she might wonder, "Wow. That was much more challenging than I could have anticipated, but I bet you could see that coming. I wonder if you wanted me to see how difficult you have had it?" Most likely, there had been an unconscious wish for the consultant to fail in order to justify their surrender. This interpretation improves communication through directness and translation of behavior. Identifying the meaning in behavior and responding with empathy and understanding demonstrate the approach to children's behavior that we hope to promote. By failing to notice this underlying communication, the consultant risks squandering the opportunity for staff to build trust in her and faith in consultation. Of course, this knowledge is not immediately apparent and requires the ability to consider one's own reactions and interactions even in the most chaotic and intense situations.

Sometimes feelings can be expressed directly but contain more subtle underlying meaning. Because consultants are often asking providers to consider the most challenging aspects of their work, they can fall victim to the providers' anger and frustration. Consequently, two challenges face the consultant: (a) handling these surface emotions without responding in kind and (b) helping caregivers explore the underlying meaning. Uncovering the feelings that lie below those expressed lessens both challenges. Sadness, isolation, lack of control, and helplessness are all emotions that confront providers as they face the needs of children and the demands of their work. Although not an extensive or thorough list, it does include those emotions that are cultural anathemas. We have all built up defenses to protect us from the fallout of these feelings. Considering them may be frightening because people imagine that these feelings are endless and all-consuming. Beginning with the children's experience may create avenues for illustrating this concept. For example, a child missing her mother wails mournfully. Anticipating that comfort will bring no consolation, the child-care provider goes about her business. Noticing the child's escalating desperation and the adult's conspicuous avoidance, the consultant addresses both by speaking for and to the child's experience: "It must be so scary to suddenly be alone in an unfamiliar world and completely helpless to conjure up the person who you know could make it better. We might worry that responding will only intensify or prolong the yearning."

3. Notice and talk about the provider's strengths. At times, consultants witness children enduring extreme harshness or concerning conditions. Perhaps more directly, consultants are daunted by the challenges that they face in these situations. Looking for places to intervene, the consultant's lens is tilted toward seeing the negative and ironically exacerbates the feeling of horror. Just as we encourage caregivers to find and build on the positive attributes of young children, the same is true for consultants with the adult caregivers. Consultation becomes more effective when the consultant can appreciate the skills and uniqueness of the caregivers. All of us are more open when we feel that we are liked and valued. Even though this seems obvious to anyone who works with children, surprisingly these tenets are abandoned frequently due to the pressure to create immediate change. Once accepted, the consultant looks for and gives voice to a provider's positive attributes.

4. Find a common goal. When consultants enter a program, they may identify areas that they wish would improve. Often the child-care providers have different goals or focus. The consultant must find the intersection of these objectives and find places for collaboration. Before that becomes possible, the consultant must inquire about the areas that the providers feel deserve consideration. What have they identified as the work "problem?" Remembering that the consultee sets the agenda bolsters the efforts to collaborate.

One program requests a consultant to help them better understand a child who "misbehaves" and is unable to contain himself. They want to know how to "discipline him more effectively." On her first visit to meet the staff, the consultant walks into a room in which the children are whirling around aimlessly. Most never light on anything for more than a moment. The first thing she notices is the lack of organization and options. All the shelves, toys, and activity opportunities are pushed against the wall creating a cavernous space that invites chaos and leaves little room for real exploration or engagement. Although their foci are different, the staff and consultant have an easy place for collaboration. Shifts in the environment will likely have immediate impact on the experience of the identified child.

Some exploration about the identified child—for instance, when and where the "misbehavior" occurs and where it is similar to the behavior of the group as a whole—might lead providers to think about the environment and create their own solutions, but staff are not always patient enough for this in a seeming crisis. The consultant, therefore, might be more direct, "It does seem that this child is having difficulty. He almost seems overwhelmed. I think some structural shifts in the environment could make his and your life easier. Would you be willing to think about making a few changes in the physical space?" The consultant accepts their view and expands on it, offering possible success with the child to relieve them of feeling so overworked. The focus of the consultant may be different from the provider's, but their common and agreed-upon goals direct their efforts. In this instance, the consultant has invested the staff in her plan to rearrange the classroom. Of course, there may be other influences that impede agreements. For instance, room arrangement may be influenced by their philosophy of child care; functional considerations, like the ease of set-up and clean-up or the ability to see all the children at the same time; and the lack of agreement among staff on arrangement, among others. All have to be considered, and the consultant has to be willing to shift course to achieve a mutual agenda.

5. *Suspend judgment.* Each consultant has their own ideals about the best care for children. Not only do approaches vary, but some child-care programs, despite valiant efforts, are unable to provide quality care. Consultants entering these programs are met with their biggest challenge: suspending judgment. A consultant does not abandon her ideals or her opinions. In order to genuinely understand a provider's perspective, a consultant must be able to listen and respond without critique. The consultant's trust in the provider's perspective makes the consultation relationship possible. Consultants may struggle to refine their language to reflect trust in the provider's view of a situation, but sometimes her choice of words may inadvertently suggest or even reveal judgment.

Those who work with children readily accept that language is powerful. The ways that consultants phrase their inquiry or idea will predict their effectiveness. Sometimes the language itself can inadvertently convey criticism, making people defensive even when the attempt is to understand.

Consider the ubiquitous question asked of young children: "Why did you do that?" Rarely does this elicit more understanding. Instead children shut down, creating more struggle in identifying intention. The same is true for adults. "Why" questions should be used sparingly because they are often experienced as critical. Phrasing the same questions with "how" or "what" will elicit more open-ended responses. For instance: How did you create the staffing schedule? What do you hope children will take away from circle time? These questions wonder about the process rather than require an answer, returning to the fundamentals of our consultation stance.

6. Avoid being the expert. Another guiding principle of consultation is to avoid being the expert. People rarely make changes in which they are not invested. The consultant's language and attitude reflect the desire to establish common ground—a place in which both parties' contributions can be made and mutual understanding developed. Becoming the expert makes it more difficult to discover these junctions. Although the role of expert can be foisted on the unsuspecting consultant, the consultant can unconsciously play the part through her actions as well as her words. The primary language tool should be the question—conveying a sense of wondering and discovery. How did you come to know that? What do you think? How have you addressed this in the past? What has worked?

By asking, the consultant reminds herself that the consultee (provider or parent) is the holder of necessary information. This does not mean that the consultant stays mute or has no knowledge to offer. Rather she reserves her "expert" advice and general knowledge until a place is readied for it to take hold. In the context of a mutual endeavor and understanding, the consultant's expertise makes its rightful contribution.

7. Convey the idea that understanding does not necessarily mean more work. Child-care providers may resist exploration that results in understanding because the process is too slow and the outcome may mean more work or responsibility. "If I know a child's history and his level of need, I must respond to all of it." In an effort to keep this awareness at bay, ignorance protects. This logic is flawed. The consultant helps ferret out what the provider can reasonably attend to and what is outside her realm of responsibility (i.e., "One can't rewrite a child's past or change his home, but in his hours here at child care what you do together and who you are to him matter.").

Although it is true that doing something different will initially feel like more work, usually the empathy that accompanies knowledge increases patience and reduces hopelessness, changing the perception of the effort involved. In addition, working with a child rather than against his behavior does make the work easier. A caregiver may not experience greater ease immediately, so a consultant should preface intervention ideas with a disclaimer—her intention is not to increase the providers' workload. Most likely, understanding will lead to shifts in attitudes and approach, but consultants must tread lightly.

8. *Use your own feelings and experiences.* Clinicians are trained to be as neutral as possible. This is a good beginning for consultation because we want to explore the subjective experience of all participants before burdening them with our shadow. As consultation progresses and providers' capabilities are revealed, a consultant may experiment with self-revelation. The consultant's disclosures can make it easier for the providers to expose their beliefs and feelings. By using herself as an example, the consultant can offer possible topics for exploration, illustrate the interplay between past and current experience, encourage honest exploration of emotions and mistakes, and, ultimately, demonstrate a general openness.

For instance, to illustrate the interlocking nature of adults' childhood experience with their current caregiving practices, a consultant might admit, "I know that when I've led groups with small children, I've counted to 10 to get the children to respond. One day I realized that the children complied because they were afraid of what might come at 10. Although I had no intention of spanking any child, deep down I knew that that was what would have happened to me as a child when my parents reached 10, and many of these children had experienced the same. Without anticipating it or consciously intending it, but reaping the benefits of it, I was using fear to control the children—the very thing I had been trying to avoid. I let my anger and frustration get the best of me. Of course, I still get angry, but I try to think twice before I count to 10. And when I absolutely can't avoid it because I'm overwhelmed, I let the children know what will come at the end of 10. I'll be the first to admit that it is nowhere as immediately effective as the ambiguous threat, but at least it's more in line with my intentions." Sometimes the providers need to know that the consultant has similar frustrations and shortcomings. Disclosure creates camaraderie and shows the consultant's willingness to accept and understand the provider's foibles, which are usually more terrifying to her than they are to the consultant.

Beyond the sharing of emotionss that echo providers' experience, the consultant must be aware of additional layers of feelings that might reveal a provider's deeper intentions. The consultant uses her own responses as a barometer. Countertransference can give clues to the provider's motivations, but it might also expose the consultant's characteristic way of responding to internal conflicts, which may interfere with the consultation process. For example, a consultant may increasingly exert control, an ingrained response to feeling powerless. She becomes demanding and takes over, ultimately blocking her intentions to collaborate with the provider. With a supervisor's help, the consultant might better use these reignited feelings of helplessness to better understand the provider rather than acting out. Identifying these motivations helps to choose language and timing of interventions. The consultant may ask herself, "What makes this important? What contributes to my response?" Using one's own feelings and responses offers insight into the consultee's experience. Understanding, rather than acting upon this information, propels the consultative process forward. When consultation is just beginning the consultant may feel a rush to attack all problems, but consultation is a longer process, taking time to accomplish goals.

Case Example

Following our own advice, we will continue to share experiences culled from our own consultation. We return to Bread and Jam Child Care after the first few months of consultation. Marsha, the consultant, has been meeting weekly with the preschool staff. A case consultation around Leo was already underway, but we will not focus on this component here. Other general program issues have emerged, including head teacher Stacey's relationship with her coworkers and discrepancies among staff in their views of hierarchy and responsibility. Although dealt with in consultation, these concerns were not voiced overtly. Instead, Marsha found these dilemmas in the content of program practices: small group, naptime, and circle time.

Marsha continues to formulate hypotheses and to understand the subjective experience of the staff. Observing their behavior with the children and each other, she will find places to enter and to intervene. By immersing herself in the relationships of the classroom, she promotes a process that in turn transforms the children's experience. We rejoin Marsha as she struggles within the strained staff dynamics and attempts to address these issues through conversations around the practical and concrete aspects of the program, such as circle time.

> Stacey, the head teacher, had requested some time alone with Marsha. What would a separate meeting mean to the others? Marsha had agreed but was nervous about the prospect of speaking with Stacey solo. She had now forged a delicate alliance with each staff member, and she did not want to jeopardize the balance by giving the appearance of siding with Stacey.
>
> Marsha had seen enough to hypothesize with her supervisor about Stacey's motivations. Status and appearing knowledgeable were extremely important. Marsha would be careful to be respectful, but avoiding colluding with Stacey's wish to fortify the hierarchy in the classroom would be challenging. Predicting her behavior and theorizing about her prior experiences, Marsha and her supervisor hoped to better navigate program consultation with her and the rest.
>
> To respect the director's (Patricia's) role, Marsha again met with her prior to her individual meeting with Stacey. Marsha and Patricia agreed that Marsha could raise questions about program practices without making them work

performance issues. However, before proceeding Marsha wanted Patricia to identify areas for improvement. Many of them paralleled Marsha's concerns but had more weight when the director voiced them. Patricia saw Stacey's strength but felt that she did not include her staff in the planning and was a bit imperious. She also worried that Leticia, who was often harsh with the children, was lazy and avoided doing work and that Harold didn't contribute as much as he should in the classroom. Their behavior became particularly troublesome during Stacey's absences because neither took responsibility for the class, leaving the planning and teaching to the substitute head teacher. Marsha wondered whether these observations were connected. Perhaps their reluctance to contribute fully resulted from the role that Stacey had assigned them. Patricia hadn't thought about that before.

Marsha wondered how Patricia had tried to help Stacey with this in the past. Patricia admitted that she avoided supervising Stacey because they had been colleagues in their student teaching days. Although they had gotten along then, things had been somewhat tense since they had reunited as supervisor and staff member. Patricia did not want to push too hard because she depended on Stacey, who was her most industrious and well-educated teacher. Yet there were moments when she wished to challenge Stacey's practices, including the marathon circle time. "I know she knows better," Patricia said with frustration. She and Marsha had agreed that Stacey was a talented teacher who had wonderful curriculum ideas. "Perhaps," Marsha theorized, "her wish to be seen as a good teacher gets in the way of seeing the children's needs and capabilities. She doesn't always feel as adept as we see her." New to their own jobs and feeling somewhat uncertain, both felt some empathy for Stacey.

Because Patricia seemed to be so understanding, Marsha thought about including her in her meeting with Stacey, but this might be premature. Although Patricia knew about their meeting, she and Marsha had agreed that Stacey might find her presence too threatening initially. Because Marsha and Patricia agreed on some of the areas for consideration, Marsha wondered if it might be helpful if she could convey some of these ideas to

Stacey with the idea that eventually Marsha would help them speak directly with one another. Patricia welcomed the help because she wanted to be more effective as Stacey's supervisor.

Despite the fact that she had requested this meeting, Stacey was late again. Marsha waited alone. Finally, Marsha tracked Stacey down, fighting down her own annoyance at Stacey's seeming lack of respect for her time. (In supervision, as she faced her own insecurities and worries about being respected, Marsha was able to better understand Stacey's behavior as a reflection of her own uncertainty rather than an indictment of Marsha's value as a consultant. For now, however, Marsha struggled to be patient.) Stacey apologized for her lateness saying that the class just couldn't function without her. Marsha said, "That's probably true. It seems like you take charge of everything. That's a lot of work." Stacey agreed.

Before meeting with Stacey, Marsha assesses the system in which they function. In this assessment, she uses her interactions with Stacey, her previous observations of the staff, Patricia's responses to her questions, and her own emotional reactions. The information reveals Stacey's internal experience, her relationship with her coworkers, and the official and unofficial hierarchy. These shape Marsha's movements. Including Patricia in the discussion, she weighs the risks and benefits of meeting with Stacey. She preserves Patricia's role as supervisor and establishes her respect for that role. She also manages to share her thought process about Stacey's choices, embodying an openness that considers not only the administrative tasks but also their emotional impact and meaning for all participants. Marsha's transparency will help Patricia develop her supervisory skills before they tackle this task directly. Consultation occurs in the interactions rather than in the exchange of concrete information.

Lateness seems to be the perennial pet peeve of consultation. As here, most people have an explanation for their tardiness. The consultant need not stop there. Even if she doesn't address it directly, she looks for underlying meaning. The consultant has to have enough experience with the program to parse out the programmatic from the personal. Marsha can see that Stacey's actions comment on their relationship, but she does not yet share this interpretation. She does use it to work more effectively with Stacey. With familiarity and permission, the consultant can raise the underlying issues as she might in therapy. She might say, "I know that you have so many things to do, but I was wondering if you're late for another reason. Perhaps, it is hard to imagine the usefulness of our meeting. I would really like to know if that is true so that we can make our meeting more constructive."

> Stacey went on to explain how she wished that the staff would take more responsibility in the classroom. "When I'm not here, it just falls apart." Marsha wondered what she made of that. Realizing that Patricia agreed with this assessment, Marsha thought that this might be an opportunity to insert the director's perspective while validating Stacey. She adds, "Patricia also worries about your absences because the class works so well when you are there, but Leticia and Harold seem to lose steam without you, leaving decisions and leadership to the substitute teacher. The children look to them for guidance, but Harold and Leticia avoid taking leadership roles. I wonder if the children become confused and anxious, making the classroom feel chaotic?" By wishing to relieve some of Stacey's pressure and by noting the stress on the children, Marsha underlined the importance of shifting this dynamic and improving the staff's skills. The emphasis placed on Stacey's great amount of responsibility appreciates her commitment to the program while also opening a window for future exploration of her contribution to the dilemma.

Although a small component of this interaction and certainly not the primary focus, the consultant introduces the idea of another's subjective experience, the voice of the director, Patricia. Because it confirms Stacey's sense of the situation, it is a relatively safe introduction. However, it is still made with careful consideration. Marsha has already received permission from Patricia to speak for her on this subject. In consideration of Stacey, she voices someone else's concerns gingerly. The consultant has shared information from another individual from a different forum. Stacey may wonder if the information that she reveals will be shared in other settings and needs reassurance that it will not be shared without permission. Despite the benign nature of the comment that Marsha shared, she will have to inquire about Stacey's response to the information as well as to the experience of the consultant's holding information between individuals. Although all participants have the right to privacy, the consultant encourages the sharing of information as the place where shifts can occur. When it is not possible, she holds information sharing as a guiding premise although never at the expense of someone's feelings of safety.

> Because Stacey's role as leader is crucial to her sense of self, Marsha hopes that Stacey will identify content issues for discussion, introducing a starting point. However, Stacey remains focused on the faults of her staff and the frustration of Leo. Marsha has more specific concerns about the classroom to which Patricia has agreed—circle time is too lengthy, naptime is too chaotic, and small groups are poorly planned and do not include all the children. Marsha begins to weave these various issues together—Stacey's staff concerns, Leo's difficulties, and Patricia's concerns about routines—"It seems important to you that the staff take more responsibility in the classroom. I imagine they need help building their skills and more encouragement. It seems like they have gotten used to taking a back seat. What do you think?" Stacey again suggests their inherent laziness, but Marsha wonders, "Do you think some of your strengths in the classroom might be seen by the others as areas they should avoid because they wouldn't do them as well? You are so competent in many ways—you carry out a circle time for longer than most are capable of doing. I imagine the others might be intimidated to try."

Marsha allows Stacey to take the lead, but she does not abandon her ideas. She attempts to find common goals and listens for the underlying message. She can respond to Stacey's insecurities while speculating about the staff's experience. She is genuinely able to commend Stacey's skills. Having communicated an authentic complement, the consultant can introduce the possible obverse effects of Stacey's competence on the rest of the staff. Without yet shifting Stacey's view of herself as a teacher, Marsha has offered another, more compassionate reason for the staff's behavior and introduced a new area for consideration: circle time.

Stacey reminded herself that circle times weren't supposed to be so lengthy but that she liked doing them. Quickly protecting herself, she reminds Marsha that most of the children are able to participate for the full time. Marsha accepts this reply but expands Stacey's consideration by adding, "The children's ability to attend is surely a sign of a successful circle time. What are some of the other hopes you have for children's participation? What do you or the other staff members see as the purpose of circle time? I'm asking because I imagine the goals inform the practice." Stacey has to contemplate the question. She hadn't ever thought about what she hoped children would learn. After a minute she begins speaking of developing greater self-control, gaining a love of stories, and forming group cohesion. Getting nervous, she begins to justify her circle time, citing pressures to prepare children for school from parents and the school district. Marsha commiserates, recognizing that sometimes external pressures and internal pulls can cause even the best intentioned to overlook what we want for children. She wonders if this topic—why we have circle time—would be a good one to discuss among all the staff. Marsha again explains her reasoning: "If we hear everybody's ideas we can start to see if there is agreement…I also imagine that Leticia and Harold need to know why they're doing something before they can do it. So this might be a way of getting them interested and more involved in participating in the way that you hope."

In Marsha's next meeting with the director, she and Patricia map out a strategy to include the other team members. Stacey's role of importance insured her participation in encouraging her team. In these early negotiations, Patricia confides her exasperation with Stacey to Marsha, who helps her to appreciate Stacey's perspective. Because Stacey and Patricia had been colleagues for years prior to arriving at Bread and Jam, Stacey struggled with their new roles in addition to her need to be seen as competent. Patricia's shakiness in her new position in management helped her to understand the dynamic because she found herself seeking Marsha's approval. Luckily for Marsha, Patricia was able to talk about her own feelings, giving Marsha the opportunity to respond empathically and to use those feelings to cultivate Patricia's empathy and understanding for her staff's difficulties.

Periodically, Marsha checked in to see what their individual meetings were like for Patricia. One afternoon after feeling particularly supported by Marsha, Patricia admitted, "Actually, I sometimes avoid meeting with you." Encouraging further revelation, Marsha wondered, "Sometimes it seems too hard?" Patricia, stammering, continued, "It's not that I don't like talking with you or that I don't find it useful." Worried that Patricia would try to take care of her rather than be honest about her feelings, Marsha interrupted, "It's hard to tell me how you feel about our meetings. It makes you somewhat anxious." "Well as a matter of fact, that's why I don't want to meet with you sometimes. I worry that you're going to think I'm incompetent," Patricia admitted. Marsha empathized, "Wow, no wonder it's difficult. Is there something that I've done to make you feel that way?" Patricia denied that Marsha had done anything. Surprising Marsha, Patricia revealed that she felt the same nervousness when she called her mother. She began to talk about her critical but absent mother. Marsha empathized and explored until Patricia's silence signaled the need for a shift. Following Patricia's lead, Marsha brought them back to the present, suggesting a similarity between Patricia's nervousness with authority and the possibility of Stacey's. This was new to Patricia, who rarely thought of herself as an authority figure, especially to Stacey. Because Patricia seemed comfortable, Marsha admitted, "It's funny how that is. I don't think of myself as an authority figure and yet you experience me that way." Patricia laughed and nodded—recognition of a growing understanding of Stacey and greater closeness with Marsha.

Marsha has found a focus for their process. Stacey, Patricia, and Marsha are invested in circle time as content through which to explore many levels of influence—the interpersonal and intrapsychic among them. Marsha hopes to help address the lengthy circle time for the children, but more importantly she wants to aid the relationships and communication among the staff members. The content makes the process more palatable to the staff. Conversely, Marsha's focus on process makes addressing the content—circle time—possible. By wondering about each provider's current experience of circle time, their positions in relation to one another, and the meaning of shared responsibility, Marsha creates an opportunity to address the particulars of practice. This inclusion addresses

Stacey's complaints of being overburdened and the other staff's "laziness." Patricia and Marsha agree that a shift in the staff relationships is necessary for the success of the classroom in Stacey's absence and for improving the children's experience.

Patricia's ability to share her own feelings will be key to the success of this consultation. Those who are more easily able to identify their feelings are usually more often able to understand and appreciate the feelings of others. In order to explore the intrapsychic experience of the staff, Marsha had to look for the first person who would let her in. Patricia's position of power makes her an important ally in this endeavor. Her ability to self-reflect will not only make her more accepting and aware of her colleagues' challenges, creating an environment that supports exploration but will offer a prototype of possibility. With practice, she may be more likely to share her process and encourage others. Furthermore, her championing this process will be more effective than Marsha's encouragement because Patricia will speak from recent experience about her own shifts, made more significant by her role as director. Marsha's assurances that self-exploration might be useful in the face of possibly painful or previously unvisited territory would be met by skepticism because the relief that she promises is as yet in the abstract. Patricia has just experienced it.

With Patricia, Marsha is careful not to delve further than she has been given permission. Marsha provides a supportive environment in which to explore. Patricia takes the path back to her past not because Marsha has directed her but because she has created the opportunity to wonder about motivations. Marsha maintains the boundary of consultation by bringing this understanding back to current circumstances to understand better adult or adult–child relationships. Although Marsha may privately call on Patricia's history when it seems to be affecting some observed interaction, she will not invite further exploration of her history unless Patricia spontaneously offers. The consultant links each new revelation back to the professional activity that prompted it.

Before revisiting Bread and Jam, let us look at all of the levels of influence at play so far in just one classroom routine—circle time. The consultant surmises that

Stacey's insecurities may stem from a lack of approval and acceptance predating her present position. These narcissistic nicks have affected her behavior and thus her relationships. Marsha won't know the particulars until much later in consultation, but she is already creating hypotheses and confirming, refuting, and changing them as she gathers more information. Stacey performs heroically during circle time to assuage her self-doubt. This one sphere of influence—*personal experience*—interacts with and influences many of the other spheres delineated earlier.

This teacher's need to achieve intersects strongly with the mandates to prepare children for kindergarten, a reflection of the *bureaucratic and government influences*. Despite Stacey's knowledge of child development, which is extensive, this need to meet others' expectations (for example, kindergarten teachers and standardized testing) permits her to disregard the actual developmental abilities of preschool children. Government guidelines quietly enter the circle. Another set of influences also intervenes here. Fearful that their children will not succeed, *parents and the community* support the force-feeding method of learning that Stacey sometimes uses. She also attempts to reinforce the established hierarchy in the realm of the *bureaucratic sphere of influence*, to which she rigidly clings for personal reasons. She sets the bar too high for others to achieve so that her role is solidified and unchallenged. Within this mix, the *staff's interpersonal relationships* (another sphere of influence) affect and are affected by these other spheres. Because her experience of self interferes with her ability to value others, Stacey sabotages efforts, her own and others', to share the burden. In response to their exclusion, the other staff members give up. They have come to share Stacey's view that she can do most things better than they can. The reasons for their relinquishing their roles may be related to each one's sense of self, but the expression is particular to these relationships. The consultant must keep each of these levels of influence in mind as she asks, explores, and advises. She has become familiar with the spheres of influence through her questions as well as her observations.

> Before the next staff meeting, Stacey and Patricia, now collaborating, had agreed that they would focus on strategies for dealing with Leo while they and Marsha moved toward the teaching staff's full participation. Stacey was

on time to the staff meeting. (Throughout the consultation, Stacey's approach to attendance revealed her current level of investment.) As planned, Patricia began the meeting by expressing her hope to better understand Leo's experience. Stacey started off by acknowledging a slight improvement in his behavior and Harold's ability to refocus Leo. Harold, who pulled his chair a little closer, smiled. Marsha asked for everyone's explanations about how Harold's help was making a difference and wondered if there were times it was more or less effective.

The staff moved quickly to the frustrations. Circle time and naptime were still a challenge. Stacey did not seem ready yet to consider circle time so Marsha began earlier, "What do you think Leo's morning is like before he gets here?" They didn't know because his mother rushed out so quickly. Marsha noted how frustrating that must be for them but gently inquired about their efforts to include her, "It's so busy in the morning, it must be difficult to greet everyone. I noticed that when I just wanted to introduce myself, Leo's mother immediately rejected me. Do you get that too?" Her admission allowed others to think about it. Soon, Patricia was wondering if they could make it a point to greet the parents. Leticia responded that they were so busy in the morning. Marsha clarified that perhaps just looking up and saying hi to the children would be enough for most. Maybe Leo and his mother needed a little more help. She made the link to Leo's entrance and how she had observed him wandering around trying to engage other children. She reminded the group how Harold had to corral Leo even in small group activities that were led by a teacher. Stacey picked this up and asked Harold to take responsibility for Leo's entrance. He quietly agreed to help Leo play with some of the other children and to greet his mother. Everyone, including Leo's mother, knew that Harold was his favorite. As they discussed the particulars, Leticia did not want to be left out, offering to greet other parents and children as they entered.

Stacey's inclusion in the decision-making process allows her to support Harold's growth. She can acknowledge his special skills and pass responsibility on to him because Marsha has done the same for her. Marsha's careful observation of Stacey as an individual and her place in the world of Bread and Jam allowed her to address Stacey's needs before she asked her to respond to Harold's. Parallel process is not just for children. The subtle shift in staff dynamics unbalances Leticia's position, and she jockeys to find a new place to maintain equilibrium. By focusing on Leo, Marsha limits the intensity of interactions but manages to address the underlying conflict. She hopes to alter the adults' relationships by encouraging process through safe content. Despite their resistances, people will begin to shift as they band together to tackle a limited problem. A consultant must find, define, and limit those goals to increase the level of safety and the hope of encouraging small successes.

Marsha had found a path: following Leo through the day. Now, at circle time, she wondered about how he was doing since her observation. Leticia complained that Leo seemed to struggle throughout, always trying to "get up close by Stacey." "What do you make of his behavior?" questioned Marsha. The group was silent. "You know, I noticed that he always seems to want to touch people. Have you noticed that too?" Marsha offered. Excitedly they agreed, pointing out how often he sucked his thumb while he pushed up against people. Marsha helped them to connect Leo's need for tactile and emotional contact to his behavior and interpreted his experience of relationships. Suddenly seeing the underlying need, not just the behavior, Leticia wished she could do more for him. Marsha suggested sitting with him in the group. Leticia's presence in the circle might make him feel more supported, literally and figuratively. Together they had created a motivation for Leticia's participation in the group rather than her usual management from a distance. This would benefit all the children. Stacey still seemed protective of her circle time so Marsha did not press on this issue. There were other meetings.

These changes, however, did not stop Marsha from feeling that she had not accomplished as much as she had hoped. Returning to supervision, she complained that circle time would remain taxing for Leo as well as the other children. Her supervisor wondered how the teachers felt about consultation. As Marsha pondered their experience, she brightened for she realized that each had felt heard and had experienced a sense of agency. Even Leticia and Harold, who had often backed away, were involved in the solution. The supervisor suggested that perhaps Leticia's presence in the circle might bring the problems to the forefront. Even with Leticia containing Leo and offering another set of hands and eyes for the other children, the group unrest would likely persist. Stacey might have to consider the effects of the circle time length on all the children.

One of the consultant's greatest tools for change is the ability to understand and voice the subjective experience of all involved. In the staff meeting, Leo was not present, and Marsha endeavors to bring greater attention to his plight. She does not, however, lecture. She wonders with staff members who bring great insight to his experience—insight that has been constricted by time constraints, responsibility for many children, and fears of additional work. Marsha creates the time by valuing staff meetings for discussion of individual children and program issues. In the last couple of months, she offered each staff member her compassion, which has now grown enough in each of them to allow them to offer the same empathy to Leo. Even though Stacey, Harold, and Leticia have not outwardly acknowledged this shift, Marsha has anticipated these results without naming each step of the process. The fact that she does not immediately reveal her assessment of Leo makes room for each of the staff to discover him through their own lens. Her thoughtfulness has fostered the staff's investment and their sense of agency. Even when one "knows," wondering can be a powerful instrument.

We have included Marsha's experience in supervision because she too becomes overwhelmed by the daunting task of helping providers consider their visions for children in their program. Every consultant needs support as well as the time and a place to consider her feelings and the meaning of interactions. Feelings of impatience arise because the pace of consultation is slow. There are too many teachers and children to consider everyone at every moment. Slowing down to wonder is essential.

Back at Bread and Jam, Patricia raised her own feelings of frustration with the sluggish pace. Using her recently acquired equanimity, Marsha helped Patricia consider the strides already made before they set goals for the next meeting. Wanting to empathize with her but also wanting to avoid discouraging her, Marsha debated whether to share her own impatience. Instead, she wondered to herself whether her wish to reveal her own frustrations would relieve Patricia or burden her with taking on Marsha's experience.

She decides to offer a more general observation, "Change often takes longer than any of us would wish." Relieved, Patricia begins to talk about how she had felt like she wasn't doing enough as the site director. "It seems like there is a lot of that going around, I bet Stacey feels the same way," Marsha adds. Patricia agrees, adding that she probably should share with Stacey how much she depends on her.

This interaction confirms the value of Marsha's supervision. With careful consideration, she uses her own experience without revealing it. Supervision allows her to contain her frustration. Because she has understood her own feelings, she is better able to use her feelings to educate and to empathize. Although personal revelations can be useful, they should be used sparingly and judiciously.

At the staff meeting, the group settled in quickly because they wanted to share their successes. Leo had been doing better. Leticia offered that she had thought for sure the other children would be jealous of the special attention Leo required, but most seemed not to notice, "He really stays right by me, if I sit with him in the group." Stacey acknowledged how helpful Leticia's participation in circle time had been. Harold noted that Leo's mother lingers a little bit in the classroom since they have been able to engage her. Harold observed, "I've been hearing how Leo's morning is going, which helps me figure out where I should get him started." Because he had the most satisfying interactions with Leo, Harold had the greatest opportunity to share positive anecdotes with Leo's mother and gain her trust. Marsha praised their successes and wondered what they made of the changes. Confidently,

Leticia explained, "He just needed to know that we cared about him and could handle him."

The shifts in the classroom had not been discussed directly, yet the accommodations to Leo eventually spilled into other programmatic arenas. General relief in the classroom, new efficacy in addressing children's challenges, and the emergence of similar issues in other children, just as Leo's were resolving, allowed for—and sometimes called for—consideration of other contributors to the classroom's conundrums. Giving Leo the responsiveness he needed during circle time had calmed the classroom, but after the 30-minute mark circle time was still challenging for most of the children.

Leticia inadvertently created an opening for Marsha, "Now that I'm not standing outside the circle, I can't see what the children are doing so easily. They are getting out of hand." "Really, do you think it has gotten worse?" Marsha queried. Stacey cringed, "I don't think so." Sensing the edge in Stacey's voice, Marsha interjected, "I wonder if you just have the time to notice more now that Leo doesn't take up all your energy." Leticia was surprised. She hadn't considered this. Stacey relaxed and Marsha asked the group, "Could something else be contributing to the difficulty? Stacey's groups are so engaging." Feeling a little safer than usual, Stacey admitted, "Well, given what I have to cover, circle time can get a little long." Leticia welcomed the opportunity to shift the power momentarily, "A little! My whole body falls asleep during your marathon circle times. I can barely get up from the floor when you are done." Stacey bristled and became defensive, "Well, they need to be prepared for kindergarten."

Marsha jumped in, "I bet you have many goals for circle time. Perhaps it would be useful if you helped Leticia and Harold understand your thinking. Your reasons for circle time may be different from theirs." Stacey felt that the calendar activities and instruction sections of her circle time were essential academic preparation. She said that the children needed to be able to sit still and listen if they were going to be ready for kindergarten, so the story time was indispensable. Of course, the greetings and songs were important for social growth. Marsha observed, "Wow, that's a lot to pack into a circle time. I'm amazed at all you can accomplish." Leticia wanted a say too: "Most of all they need to listen." Marsha clarified, "Stacey wants them to have that practice too, but that seems particularly important to you." Leticia insisted that it was important for the children to respect adults when they are talking: "That's why I used to make sure that everyone was paying attention." Marsha added, "I remember, it upset you when they looked like they weren't listening. Is it easier now that you have been focused on Leo?" "No, now I can't keep everyone in line," Leticia responded. "My guess is that children's respecting adults is important to all of us, but we might differ in what we think respect looks like," Marsha offered. Leticia became somewhat angry, "When I was young, you would get whipped if you didn't act right." Trying to show understanding, Marsha said, "No wonder this is so important to you, it sounds like it was the number one rule in your family." Waiting a moment, she added, "What we've learned in our families is always important. I think it can be hard when people have different ideas or experiences. I agree that listening to adults is important. I have some thoughts about this. Would it be okay if I shared them?" Leticia nodded affirmatively, and the rest of the group appreciated the shift as Marsha continued, "Child care can be a stress on children and adults. All these adults and children bring their varied experiences and expectations with them. When they are different, it can be hard to feel like what you believe in is valued. Add to this that little ones learn through their bodies as well as through their brains." Leticia seemed ready to argue, but Marsha pushed on a little bit more, "I know, some of the children are completely capable of sitting through circle time, but not all of them are there yet. I think the fact that Stacey's circle times are so engaging has masked the range of abilities." Stacey jumped in, "I know this." Marsha's indicating, "Of course," encouraged Stacey to go on, "I push the children so that we have time to include all the important stuff. There is no way that I could squeeze it all in otherwise." "See," Leticia nodded emphatically to Marsha.

Stacey interrupted her, "Although I have to say, Leticia, that I think circle time is a lot easier now that you are in it than when you watched from outside." "So, Leticia, it sounds like your involvement is a benefit to everyone, but you see it as shirking your responsibility to instill respect?" asked Marsha. This surprised Leticia, who thought that she should do more to discipline the children. Stacey laughed, "I want you to do more, but not more yelling." Having discussed this with Stacey previously and wanting to encourage rather than cut off dialogue, Marsha added, "I think Stacey is saying your participation is an asset and even more powerful than policing from the sidelines." Stacey caught on and added, "I wish sometimes that you would do more of the singing activities because you have such a nice voice and the children pay attention more when you join in."

With Marsha's encouragement, Leticia expressed her worries, "If I act like one of the children, they won't respect me or listen to me." "No wonder it has been difficult to join in. I think Stacey is suggesting the children actually follow your direction better when they see, rather than hear, what you expect. But I don't know if imitating you feels like a form of respect. I don't think either of us realized that you weren't feeling respected," said Marsha, "I imagine you were trying to tell us that earlier when you wanted the children to listen. I suspect that this is one of those differences that can sometimes make communication difficult. We all have different ideas based on our family and cultural experiences." Leticia added, "And age. I guess I am also from a different generation." Things seemed to relax a bit as Stacey explained why Leticia's presence in the group was important on a daily basis and for preparation for the days when Stacey is out. Trying to reassure Leticia, Marsha asked, "Have you had trouble leading the children since you've been participating in the group?" "Well, actually no," admitted Leticia. Marsha clarified, "I think the children are able to see the difference between your participating and being another child. Sometimes when children feel closer to someone, they are actually more apt to follow their directions. I think that is what has happened for Leo and most likely will happen for the rest of the children." Not quite ready to leave this, Marsha asked Stacey how Leticia could be helpful in the group. For the first time, Stacey was willing to turn over orchestration of the singing to Leticia because she resonated with the worry about not being respected. Leticia seemed to like this idea.

Marsha wanted to ensure its success so she warned that the change in leadership might be an adjustment for the children. She ended, "Perhaps you might want to start with a tiny change so Leticia's contribution is noticeable but not overwhelming." Stacey seemed to think this was a good reason to shorten the group. Her new role as a mentor to her staff made showing her teaching prowess a little less important. On the days when she led the circle time alone, Stacey still stretched the time but was more careful because she was "training" Leticia.

Although the staff would have chosen to continue talking about Leo, the consultant was able to use him as a conduit to address more general issues in the circle time. The fact that she had responded to their initial concerns allowed her to move between the two. Most important, she helps them to see that their varying views of circle time actually impact their communication with each other and the functioning of the activity. Addressing the seemingly obvious, Marsha asks about the purpose of circle time. The variation reveals not only the providers' attitudes toward the activity and children but helps them to make the shift to focusing on the programmatic.

Stacey and Leticia, following the lines of hierarchy, have agreed to their relative positions without considering the effects on each of them. Stacey is burdened with responsibility, and Leticia experiences a lack of respect. By outlining these components, Marsha helps them to come to a more agreeable solution in which each feels greater effectiveness. Because the hierarchy remains important to Stacey, Marsha is careful to imbue their new roles with a similar order. Mentoring her staff allows Stacey to share control, and the new found respect gives Leticia more investment and thus greater enthusiasm for her job.

Marsha helps them to make these underlying worries and unspoken communications conscious without making them threatening. The consultant is aware of and curious about the cultural differences influencing teaching and communication styles, the varying developmental needs of the children, and the individuals' feelings about each other and children.

Leo stayed a focus of the consultation, but many aspects of the program were also addressed. Focusing on him allowed for greater participation and investment in the process that addressed the staff difficulties, classroom schedule and rules, and the individual needs of adults and children. Without imposing her child-care ideals, Marsha attempts to foster an environment that is more reflective and supportive of the teaching staff and nurturing to the children. When she first began, this combination seemed impossible to the teachers, especially Leticia. The safety of the content provided shelter from the perceived dangers of process, and the process created shifts in everyone's experience.

References

Bredekamp, S., & Copple, C. (Eds.). (1997). *Developmentally appropriate practice in early childhood programs.* Washington, DC: National Association for the Education of Young Children.

Cost, Quality and Outcomes Study Team. (1995). *Cost, quality and child outcomes in child care centers* (Technical report). Denver: University of Colorado.

Klugman, E., & Smilansky, S. (1991). *Children's play and learning: Perspectives and policy implications.* New York: Teachers College Press.

Lally, R., Griffin, A., Fenichel, E., Segal, M., Szanton, E., & Weissbourd, B. (1995). *Caring for infants and toddlers in groups: Developmentally appropriate practice.* Washington, DC: ZERO TO THREE.

Seefeldt, C. (Ed.). (1991). *The early childhood curriculum: A review of current research.* New York: Teachers College Press.

Whitebrook, M., Howes, C., & Phillips, D. (1998). *Worthy work, unlivable wages: The National Child Care Staffing Study, 1988–1997.* Washington, DC: National Center for the Early Childhood Work Force.

Whitebrook, M., Howes, C., & Phillips, D. (1989). *The National Child Care Staffing Study Who Cares? Child care teachers and the quality of care in America.* Washington, DC: National Center for the Early Childhood Work Force.

Chapter 5

Adult Relationships

An infant has trouble relaxing into sleep and resists comforting. A 3-year-old girl races around her home and rarely listens to direction. A 5-year-old boy begins to wet the bed after a year of dry nights. At these moments, after exhausting all imagined responses with little success, parents pursue outside assistance, perhaps a mental health professional: "What's wrong with my child?" As parents tell the story of the problem and the history of their child, they reveal difficulties in their relationships perhaps as a result of or prior to the difficulty. The presence of the sleep-depriving crying infant, who had not been planned, has taxed her parents beyond their tentatively brokered peace and left little room for new treaties. Occasional outbreaks of domestic violence have been followed by silent tensions. The baby has served as the only safety barrier between the two as they stay together for "her sake." In the home of the 3-year-old, her Asian-American father has insisted that his mother, who was recently widowed, move into their home despite the wishes of his wife, who is of Northern European descent. Although the grandmother warmed slightly to her daughter-in-law after the birth of her granddaughter, she has been mostly disappointed since her son married. Their newly configured home life is filled with resentment. The 5-year-old boy's father had also wet the bed as a child but, more importantly, recently left the home. His son only sees him on Saturday afternoons while the parents work out their custody arrangement. The parents may not see the connection between their challenges and their children's, but the links are unmistakable. The health of adults' relationships thoroughly affects their children's well-being.

Although these connections seem self-evident when considering parents, adult relationships are rarely considered in child care. Child-care providers don't make formal commitments to one another nor do their connections with children hold the singular significance of parenting. However, for the very reason that child-care providers are thrust with little choice into the intimate relationship of caring for children, we should look closely at these relationships and their affect on the welfare of child care's children.

Our experience and process evaluations (Pawl & Johnston, 1991) over the years have demonstrated that the quality of care is linked to the child care's organizational functioning. Those programs in which the adult relationships were ill-defined or conflictual had the lowest level of quality in the care of children. When adults don't feel understood, respected, or able to anticipate transitions, they are not likely to understand, respect, or anticipate the needs of children. This parallel is at the heart of child care and consultation.

In this chapter, we look more closely at the adult relationships that allow child care to function. We will examine the specific challenges of the child care profession requiring intimate and intense interactions, the social forces impinging on those relationships, and the individual differences contributing to miscommunication. Then, we will offer suggestions for repairing troubled relationships and improving adult communication. The same concepts will be applied to the teacher–parent affiliations as we prepare for more intense consideration of these relationships in upcoming chapters on case consultation. We will look at the consultant's position and role in the ongoing effort to improve the quality of care through attention to adult relationships. Strictly child-focused interventions may seem simpler and achieve some relief, but those that address the complexity of the adults' alliances may be most effective.

The Required Intimacy of the Child-Care Profession

In the bustling life of child care, the needs of children remain intense throughout the day. As one child finds an engaging activity, another has wet her pants or cries for a lost toy. When one scuffle is resolved between two children desperately holding on to the same shovel, another begins with the loudly uttered phrase, "I'm not your friend." One infant wakes crying for her mother just as the baby in the next crib has finally been lulled to sleep with a half hour of rocking.

Responding to these varied and changing needs can be exhausting. No adult could possibly handle the demands alone.

The internal shifts required to respond to the ever-changing moods and raw, undiluted emotions of the children require an emotional openness and an ability to handle rising stress levels. Maintaining this level of engagement with the children and with fellow providers may not always be possible, especially when there is little support, respect, or financial reward for the work. When overwhelmed, providers tend to dampen their responses to children and to their coworkers. Both can feel isolated and alone. At the other end of the spectrum, some become frustrated and short-tempered with the children and each other. When unattended, the emotional overcharge builds and leaks out in interactions with the children and often between caregivers.

Child care is also a profession that requires more sharing than most. Space, materials, and time are all in limited supply. The afternoon shift uses the same classroom and supplies after the morning team has finished with them. The way that the classroom is left in the afternoon will affect the morning staff's routine. Every aspect of the day is communal. If one person spends a few minutes more on break, her coworker's break is delayed, not to mention the fact that the very idea of a break often leaves some aspect of the program understaffed.

Juggling the day's duties has its own challenges. Who diapers, sets up for snack, or leads circle time? Usually divvied up without discussion, these jobs can carry their own burdens and resentments. Over time these slights can add up. With no time to discuss the task assignments, providers assume the responsibility consistent with their tolerance level—usually not an effective or fair distribution of duties. For instance, Mary needs to know that the trays are clean, tables are wiped, and cots are set out as soon as the children leave the room for outside time. Although her co-teacher, Yvonne, would be willing to do these tasks, she does not see the same level of urgency and would leave these chores until all the children re-entered for hand washing and toileting, leaving just enough time to hurriedly assemble for lunch and naptime and preserving the teacher–child ratio outside. Yvonne has come to resent being in the yard by herself with so many children, and Mary believes that she always has to clean up after Yvonne and the children. Even when Mary and Yvonne have agreed to shift responsibilities, Mary jumps in early because she thinks that Yvonne will never get the work done. Because Yvonne would prefer to be with the children anyway, she has accepted the status quo and lets Mary do what she wants. Unfortunately, it isn't what Mary wants but what she believes she has to do. Tension has continued to build.

Under this exchange lies another emotional barrier. Sometimes to avoid the intensity of the children's feelings and the responsibility of responding to their needs, providers can hide behind the clean-up duties. A part of Mary also avoids outside time with the children because she dislikes the loudness and mayhem of recess. Without regular breaks, her lengthy lunch and naptime preparations provide some respite. Because there has been no time to withdraw from or to discuss her stresses and the work, she remembers only the resentments and burden. Her anger might be better placed with the lack of funding for child care that leaves programs understaffed, but it is more easily and immediately vented on her coworker.

Devaluation and Child Care

The complexity of adult relationships in child care is exacerbated by the daily stressors created by the demands of child care and the lack of respect for the child- care profession. Even when people agree that raising children is an important contribution to our society, this value is rarely transferred to the profession of raising children—child care. Child-care providers internalize this devaluation and play this theme out with each other.

In addition, child care reflects this societal devaluation in many of its practical aspects. In turn, these practices ironically confirm the lack of value that society affords the child-care profession. Child-care wages are some of the lowest in our culture. Often, the wages at a fast food restaurant are more than the entry-level position in child care. Both inside and outside the child-care profession, the compensation confirms the widely held view that anyone could do it.

The scarcity also makes child-care professionals extremely sensitive to the pay differences from aide to head teacher. It is important to reward people for increased responsibility, but it can be difficult to see the reason for the pay differential when on the floor the work seems so similar.

When the work isn't deemed important, creating opportunities to talk about it hardly seems useful. As a result, many programs suffer from a lack of role clarity that brings its own resentments. Each person defines their own array of duties and unconsciously assigns the duties of others, breeding misunderstanding. Furthermore, the work of child care is extremely personal. With few opportunities (let alone scheduled time) to discuss these challenges, problems arise. Sometimes the lack of discussion time is institutionalized, reflecting the general devaluation of the child-care professionals' thoughts and feelings; schedules don't allow for any overlap between staff shifts that might encourage some exchange of information. The afternoon shift begins the same minute the morning shift ends. When there are differences in approaches and views of children and child care among staff members, the complexity of the challenges and misunderstandings expand exponentially.

Child-care professionals are oppressed, but they have no easily identifiable oppressor. Instead, their frustration and dissatisfaction are often directed at each other. Some give up entirely and just show up for work, barely contributing. Unable to acknowledge a lack of self-esteem, some project this diminished value on others, treating their coworkers or parents with little respect. This internalized devaluation is contagious and damaging. For staff members who have experienced this form of treatment in other arenas of their life, the similarities can confirm negative expectations. Entwined in these struggles for many hours of the day, they act out their internal battles with each other.

The reasons that people choose the child-care profession are varied. Some join the field because they adore and are extremely knowledgeable about children and want to be in the helping profession. Others enter the field because they don't feel equipped for other professions, and this one requires little training to begin.

On its face, child care also initially promises a profession that requires little adult interaction. Consequently, some enter the profession in the hopes, at least unconsciously, of easier, less threatening relationships. Understanding and engaging children may be more compatible with one's character. The hope of having one's goodness and competency reflected by adoring children is enthralling. Unfortunately, even when these interactions work out well with the children, the adult is surprised to find the required pressure of many adult relationships with coworkers and parents.

Of course, each staff member brings her own history and culture that has shaped her and her perceptions of the work and children. These varied experiences largely influence how she engages and views others. These differences, which are difficult to negotiate in any job, are magnified by the highly personal nature of child care. For many hours each day, people are working side by side in an extremely collaborative effort responding to the great and shifting needs of children and their families, who demand emotional availability and challenge feelings of competency. The intensity of the relationships and the pressure of child care's logistical demands force child-care professionals to face their own vulnerabilities from moment to moment and unexpectedly. The fact that most child-care programs manage this with equanimity is amazing.

The varied responses to one's own needs and those of children can create conflict among the child-care team. One teacher's wish to ignore crying children and possibly avoid the associated feelings is thwarted by her coworker who feels distress must be soothed immediately. Each bases her response on her beliefs, experiences, and tolerance for affect. When these differences begin to touch the individual's vulnerabilities and varied staff responses threaten to unbalance the program's equilibrium, conflicts and resentments can foment.

Just as in the case of battling parents, children are caught in the middle of the conflict—both acknowledged and repressed. The children's welfare is used to support both sides of the argument. At other times, the children suffer from the unexpressed feelings as the staff members' tempers rise and patience shortens.

Sometimes individual children begin to express these tensions through their behavior becoming the "identified problem." Rather than engaging each other, the providers become entangled in struggles with particular children. When the adults in children's lives support and respect each other, the children feel safer, more confident, and better able to express themselves without fear. Children's growth is dependent on the health of adult relationships.

Addressing the Adult Relationships

By the time consultants enter the child-care program or are invited to address staff difficulties, a history has developed among the staff. Entrenched views of one another are often based on assumptions. They have not been able to talk about or address their misunderstandings. Logistically and sometimes philosophically, there is little space to talk directly with one another about why they do what they do. The value of talking at all, let alone about one's experience or feelings, may not be sanctioned. Furthermore, the general lack of value for the work makes discussing it seem unnecessary. The consultant faces the task of raising the significance of any discussion in addition to sorting out the misinterpretations of each other's actions.

The consultant needs to give each person a voice—identify and share the subjective experience of each member of the child-care community—the providers, the children, and their parents. She begins by attempting to understand the reasons for each member's actions, instilling the idea that the adults' experience can and should be considered. While taking cues about the pace from the participants, the consultant builds a bridge of communication in which each member feels understood by the others.

Rarely do providers discuss their experience, past or present, in the context of child care until consultation introduces its importance. The most recent evaluation of our services (James Bowman Associates & Kagan, 2003) found that through the course of consultation the content of the staff meetings' conversations shifted from administrative negotiations to talk about the children's and adults' experience. The consultant prepares the path for this exploration.

Instilling the idea of the importance of the adult experience in child care, the consultant often begins with the director. She negotiates the schedule and content of staff meetings with her. By asking questions about the director's experience and her understanding of the staff's perceptions and experience, the consultant suggests her investment in learning the motivations and meaning of the adults' behavior as well as the children's behavior.

Initially, the consultant serves as the conduit for each person's perceptions. She validates without aligning with any one position. In the beginning, the consultees, even when in a group, may speak only directly to the consultant. She is the one inviting their opinions, and it does not yet feel safe to expose oneself to the others. The consultant, therefore, interprets and translates each person's intentions with two goals in mind. First, she is moving toward people speaking directly to one another. While recognizing that they may not be ready to do so, she is always looking for ways and opportunities for direct communication. Second, she attempts to establish a practice of communication in which members compromise in the moment and in the future. She attempts to find amicable solutions for all.

Consultant's Position

In the beginning of the consultation process, participants may speak through the consultant in meetings. The consultant looks for opportunities to open the discussion to include the others by asking others to respond or by breaking eye contact to look for other's reactions. Her shift hopes to invite the speaker to include others. At the same time, she appreciates that for the moment she may be the easiest person to speak with because she remains as neutral as possible throughout.

Although the goal is always to bring the discussion back to the group, sometimes the consultant finds it necessary to speak with members individually. Some providers may not feel safe addressing the group on the basis of past experiences or current exchanges with their colleagues. Mai-Lin's family heartedly disapproved of complaints or other expressions of emotions and would shun violators. That she was willing to do so with the consultant was a surprise for Mai-Lin, but she was not yet ready to address her coworkers. The risk of exclusion and disapproval was too great. Until the consultant had prepared the group for this level of disclosure and raised Mai-Lin's trust in her and the others to tolerate her dissatisfaction, the consultant met alone with Mai-Lin to relieve some of the pressure. Back in the group, the consultant created opportunities and raised the associated general issues, but she neither demanded Mai-Lin's participation nor spoke for her. She had not yet received permission.

At other times, individuals are overwhelmed by personal concerns that they do not wish to share with their colleagues. Myesha was wearing long sleeves because the bruises on her arm would reveal her boyfriend's abuse. Her weepiness in the classroom was concerning to everyone including the children. When the consultant arrived, Myesha couldn't contain it any longer and needed to speak with her then. The consultant empathized with her fears and offered her referrals to different services. For the moment, the consultant was the only one privy to Myesha's distress. Sharing her burden with the coworkers that she saw daily felt too shameful. With the consultant's help, however, Myesha was able to acknowledge her change in mood and the effect on her coworkers. The consultant facilitated this discussion and protected Myesha by keeping further personal questions at bay.

Confidentiality and Privacy

These private conversations raise the boundary between therapy and consultation. In therapy, the patient has the right to confidentiality in which no subject is raised with others. Consultation has different boundaries. Although the consultant always respects each person's right to privacy, her client is actually the group. The consultant needs to make this clear as she invites individual conversations. She will not discuss an individual's issues with others without permission, but she always has the goal of greater communication and understanding in the group. To that end, (a) she will encourage providers to bring up their concerns in the group; (b) she will ask permission to raise the issue herself and possibly speak for the staff member; or (c) she may broach a subject generally without identifying the person who raised the issue.

> For instance, Gloria, a teacher's assistant, has complained that sick children are allowed to enter or to remain at school despite her understanding of the policy. Her resentment has slowly built until she is snapping at the teacher, Betty, over formerly minor irritations, much to her coworker's confusion. Although Gloria has confessed anger and feelings of powerlessness to make decisions about the sick children's attendance to the consultant, she can't imagine challenging Betty. While encouraging Gloria to speak up and offering help, the consultant respects Gloria's decision not to do so. Instead, she gets approval to raise the issue in staff meeting. When Betty raises other concerns about an obviously sick child, the consultant wonders about how the child's illness may be affecting his experience in the program and later asks how decisions are made about sending sick children home. Betty acknowledges that she bends the rules because she doesn't want to overburden the parents. Feeling protected, Gloria can challenge this logic by raising concerns about the teachers' health and the health of other children. When Betty voices her reluctance to confront parents, the consultant wonders if Gloria could also speak with parents. To Gloria's surprise, Betty welcomes the help and doesn't mind the circumventing of authority. Gloria's problem is resolved without addressing the level of her frustration directly with Betty.

In the process above, the consultant has demonstrated that discussion without conflict is possible. The consultant supports and demonstrates direct communication. In time, the pattern of appropriate and satisfying exchanges encourages experimentation with and without the consultant. Privacy becomes less important as colleagues come to trust each other.

In the meantime, however, the consultant makes the distinction between confidentiality and privacy. She will not discuss the staff's challenges outside the program except with her supervisor. This conforms to traditional ideas of confidentiality, and she spells out the legal limits. Because people will be revealing aspects of their own lives that may include child abuse, elder abuse, homicidality, and suicidality, she needs to warn them in advance that information regarding those subjects will require that she share that information with appropriate authorities.

With individuals in the group, she expresses her wish to respect the individual's privacy. She will not reveal details that are not associated with the welfare of the children or the interstaff relationships, but she will endeavor to raise issues that impact those areas. Gloria had also revealed that her difficulty disagreeing with Betty was related to her own experiences with an abusive father who demanded that his word never be challenged under penalty of beatings. Although this informed the intensity and ways in which the consultant encouraged Gloria to speak directly with Betty, the consultant never revealed this information to the group. She both gained Gloria's trust and demonstrated to her the possibility of confrontation without violent repercussions. Her intervention is therapeutic without being therapy.

Working With Directors

The director is often the gatekeeper to consultation. Ultimately, it is her support that allows for exploration of interstaff issues. This means that the consultant has to establish the value of adult communication and help the director to support and facilitate it. The consultant should work toward the goal of having the director herself help the staff communicate more effectively and with her, but this is often not possible in the beginning of consultation. In the meantime, the consultant models techniques and talks about the communication process with directors.

Directors are most often promoted from within the ranks of the teaching staff. Considered a reward for work well done, the promotion may represent more money and more prestige. Again, even though the promotion may be based on the quality of work with the children, the promotion's value is established with the administrative and managerial responsibilities, inadvertently lowering the value of the child–provider relationships. Sometimes, new directors regret their move because they entered child care for the rewards of working directly with children. Unfortunately, for greater pay and perhaps greater respect, they give up their love to supervise others doing it.

Because they came up through the ranks, directors usually have little experience supervising adults. Most directors have been promoted because they were able to create a cooperative atmosphere among the children yet, ironically, this knowledge doesn't always translate to creating collaborative relationships among the adults. Sometimes, management focuses on the more practical aspects of running an organization like schedules and budgets rather than supervising adults. Although there is usually little preparation for these aspects, their concrete nature demands attention.

Attending to the adult relationships can fall by the wayside, especially when there are special challenges and little preparation. Often, the director is asked to supervise former colleagues. The shift in hierarchy can unbalance even the most supportive relationships. The director may avoid supervising altogether in these instances, ignoring problems (as in the case of Patricia and Stacey at Bread and Jam Child Care. Colleagues years before, Patricia avoided supervising or even making suggestions to Stacey for fear that she might show resentment or possibly anger). At the other end of the spectrum, the director may work too hard at establishing authority and alienate her staff.

Moving up for a job well done is an important incentive, but usually there has been little preparation for key aspects of the role. To simplify this challenge, directors may minimize the supervising aspects and focus on the more easily learned administrative tasks. If there are staff meetings, this will leak into these forums too. Staff meetings can often focus primarily on staff schedules and paperwork rather than more relationally oriented topics like shared child-care philosophy, the juggling of the classroom functioning among the adults (including satisfaction or dissatisfaction), and communication with parents.

Encouraging Communication

The consultant might encourage more regular staff meetings to balance the administrative with the interpersonal. With more time, the practical aspects are covered freeing time for the latter. Often as the consultant begins consultation with the director, the director will request help with getting staff to conform to the program's rules and guidelines. The consultant reframes this by wondering about the reasons for the resistance. While helping the director to gain control over her administrative and supervisory functions, she is helping her to imagine future preventative measures, most always addressing aspects of the relationships between the director and the staff or among the staff members.

Staff meetings are also useful as a form of communication practice. When there are no regular forums for communication, it is more difficult for staff members to speak amicably about difficulties because the conflicts are only addressed when they feel dire. Then, the grim prediction that conflict only leads to anger and separation comes true because the staff meeting is the place where people blow up. In turn, staff meetings are avoided in an attempt to avoid conflict. The consultant helps the director to see that as people feel heard they are more willing to embrace the organization's philosophy. They are contributing members of the organization.

The consultant's stance is always as neutral and nonjudgmental as possible. This can be difficult for the consultant to achieve but even more demanding for the group. When all information is at least initially accepted without moral assessments, people are more likely to share their ideas and thoughts. In the beginning, the consultant is trying to collect as much information as possible before making decisions with the group. She shares this intention with the director and with staff. The experience of being freely heard has the benefit of encouraging this type of exchange among all members of the team. However, as members feel heard and begin to feel that they have an ally in the consultant, they can also feel betrayed when she represents another, perhaps opposing, view.

To diffuse some of the judgment and possible anger toward each other, the consultant might translate for the participants. In some more extreme cases in which direct communication might only fuel anger, she might have participants speak to her before sharing ideas. As she helps to interpret one coworker's words to another, she tries to drain the judgment and diffuse the energy. She may help them to find the words or amend attitudes so their statements don't feel so accusatory. She may do this on the spot in group meetings, rephrasing a provider's comments so others might hear the underlying intention.

> When Mary and Yvonne, who were introduced earlier, finally discussed their distribution of clean-up and preparation duties, resentments obscured their wishes and intentions. Mary began one of their meetings, "I am sick and tired of doing all the work around here." Having discussed this earlier with both, seeing Yvonne's stunned shock, and wishing to help all feel heard, the consultant tempers Mary's statement, "You are really angry about taking on so many duties. I know that you have felt that you have to always clean up." Yvonne counters, "And I'm always the one who never gets a break from the kids." The consultant tries to find the commonalities, "Yvonne, it sounds like you actually would want to do some of the clean-up duties?" Mary is surprised by Yvonne's wish and willingness. "And Mary, I think you would want to spend more time with the children. You have been so quick to take on the clean-up duties that I think that I, and probably Yvonne, have assumed that you wanted to do them." As the conversation continues, the consultant tries to figure out how the current arrangement came to be. They come to understand that Mary's lower tolerance level for the undone cleaning tasks makes her assume greater responsibility. Then, they can work out arrangements that serve both better. In response to Mary's anxiety, Yvonne shifts tasks, taking on some of the cleaning duties and doing them sooner

than she might if she were alone. With the dilemmas spelled out, Mary has to examine her motivations for taking on extra clean-up duties. Sometimes, she does do more than she would like, but she also has to accept that it is in part her choice. If Mary waits long enough, Yvonne will take responsibility for clean-up. As the roles shift, Mary also has to acknowledge that she has appreciated the respite from the children that wiping tables and trays has provided. In time, Mary and Yvonne ironically return to the previous distribution of activities, but their understanding of their own and each other's motivations makes the apportionment feel more equitable.

Case Example

Because individual experiences are often more instructive than general discussions, we return to Bread and Jam Child Care. In the preceding few months, much had improved in the preschool class. Head teacher Stacey's circle time was shorter but no less lively. The dialogue that developed among the staff had encouraged the change in the routine and broadened to other topics. As a result, Leo, the child who had been having so much difficulty with the providers, was thriving and had developed close attachments to the adults who now returned the affection. Seeing the shift in both program practices and interstaff atmosphere, Patricia, the director, asks for help working with the teachers from the toddler room, Tyra and Bob. Marsha has had brief friendly interactions with both, but there been no time for staff meetings or discussion of their classroom until now. Patricia had asked the consultant to focus on the preschool class because her time was limited and the classroom's demands including Leo were greater. This was shifting.

> The crises in this classroom had abated. Leo was doing quite well with some extra help from Harold and some shifts in classroom functioning. However, by January more pressing concerns arose for Patricia in another classroom. "I really need your help with Tyra and Bob. It's gotten out of hand."

Bob and Tyra, with some support staff, shared the morning and afternoon toddler room duties respectively. Through observation and discussion with Patricia, Marsha would find Tyra to be a hard worker who made elaborate plans in perfect sync with the children. Bob was much more casual about his work, but the children found him to be a strong comforting presence who made them feel safe. Potentially, they could create the perfect team, but they had a long way to go before they could work together successfully.

Two days ago, Bob had made an inappropriate joke that, until Tyra reacted, he thought very amusing. From an older generation, he was unaware of the misogyny it contained; however, when made aware, he apologized. Tyra, however, could not be satisfied. She had written down her complaint and had presented it ceremoniously to Patricia, wanting her "to take care of it." Marsha entered here. Together they wondered what Tyra hoped might happen. "Probably fire him," admitted Patricia, "I've been avoiding this for a long time. Because they only overlap for a brief time during the day, it seemed that they could just hold on." Marsha chuckled in support, "I guess they let go."

Patricia filled Marsha in on Tyra's history—difficult peer relationships that resulted in frequent moves from one child-care center to another—as they tried to figure out what to do. As at Bread and Jam, however, she had excellent relationships with the children. It was clear that Tyra wanted Patricia's protection and that she likely felt that she worked harder than Bob. Marsha offered to meet with Patricia and Tyra to understand her concerns better. Marsha tried to anticipate possible scenarios with Patricia to prepare her for possibilities the director had been avoiding. For instance, they imagined that Tyra or Bob could become angry or shut down.

Soon after, the three met together. Angrily, Tyra turned to Marsha, "So now you meet with me." "Had you wanted to meet earlier and I hadn't made that available?" "No." Although Tyra never admitted it, she was jealous of the other classroom's opportunity to meet with Marsha. Marsha would discover later that now that things were going well in the preschool room, those staff members had shared with Tyra their enthusiasm for and relief they felt from meetings with the consultant. In the moment, however, Marsha tried hard to understand Tyra's resentment but was dumbfounded. Finally, Marsha just apologized, admitting that she hadn't realized that Tyra wanted or even needed meetings. Continuing, she tried, "You always seem so confident with the children when I've happened by the yard. I didn't realize there might be other reasons we could be meeting, but how we get along with our coworkers is equally important. I'm sorry that I didn't know our meeting could have been useful. I wish you could have let me or Patricia know rather than having to hold it all by yourself. I realize now that I should have made myself available to everyone." This calmed Tyra.

Tyra's anger illustrates how much the consultant's actions have meaning. Although Marsha had been attentive to the effects of her presence and interactions with the preschool classroom, she had not considered what those interactions might mean to others at the child-care center. Although she could not possibly have anticipated or served all the needs of the program, Marsha, now, must understand and respond to the results of her actions and inactions.

In addition, the consultant sometimes must hold the responsibility as well as the hope and possibility of change. Marsha's acknowledgement of her own blind spot acknowledges that Tyra's perceptions and experience are important to her. Her response also offers another possible type of interaction, one that Tyra's usual style prevents. Marsha's offering an apology and accepting Tyra's view gives Tyra the experience that another respects her and values her feelings. Marsha's very actions challenge Tyra's worldview and her interaction style without attacking it specifically.

Marsha tried to bring them back to the task at hand, "Patricia asked me to join so that we could understand your concerns better. Will that be useful?" "Whatever," Tyra replied curtly. With Marsha's assistance, Patricia expressed her concern, outlined how she planned to respond, and asked for Tyra's thoughts. Together they decided that Patricia would speak with Bob directly and put her expectations in writing for the entire staff. Marsha added that while the director's ideas were important, she (Marsha) imagined the relationship could be repaired only as the coworkers could reestablish trust and talk directly. In general, Tyra seemed satisfied, but she fought the meeting with Bob even though Marsha framed it as partly for his edification. Patricia professed her wish for the meeting and made the final decision. Patricia's decisiveness could be challenging, but for now Marsha was appreciative.

In their first meeting, Bob was welcoming and affable as he would be throughout consultation, but he was not nor would he ever be particularly excited about Marsha's presence. Meeting about work meant the possibility of more, which as Tyra accurately reported, he tried to avoid. Patricia voiced her concerns about the recent joke and laid out the new policy. To his credit, Bob wholeheartedly agreed and turned to Tyra and again apologized. She looked away in disgust. Marsha shared an empathic exchange with Bob signaling with her expression, "This is tough." Eventually, they moved on to discuss other aspects of the team's interactions. Tyra railroaded the conversation, reporting all her hard work, implicitly underscoring Bob's lack of contribution. Marsha and Patricia's efforts to insert some ideas, encourage Bob's input, or even praise Tyra were overridden. The hour had exhausted Marsha as well as Patricia.

At the bimonthly toddler staff meetings, Tyra overwhelmed whoever was present with descriptions of her classroom successes. Marsha struggled to facilitate rather than watch passively, but inserting a space for any of the other teachers' voices was a challenge. Patricia was becoming less and less tolerant and more and more aggravated and was threatening to end the meetings entirely. Marsha ran back and forth between Patricia and her supervisor and began to better understand Tyra. Without any encouragement from Marsha, Rosie, the school secretary, offered further clarification probably because she had been listening in on Marsha and Patricia's conversations. In her late 20s, Tyra still lived at home with her mother who, based on Rosie's experience with her in the community, was nasty and critical. Her father had abandoned Tyra at 2. They had been alone since then.

Although Marsha never would reveal this knowledge to Tyra, she reflected on it often. Her thoughts and actions with Tyra were informed by her sense that these experiences accounted, at least in part, for Tyra's exchanges with others. Patricia, who also knew, was able to empathize with the experience of a critical mother for she had spent years shedding the effects of her own similar experiences through therapy. Marsha reminded her that Tyra was at the beginning of that journey. They decided to meet with Tyra alone so that she could tell them about her successes in the classroom. Marsha offered her admiration and praise. Despite the exhaustion of these meetings, the meetings including Bob were freed for at least some negotiation of classroom activities and discussion of the children.

Although not a therapist, the consultant is always aware of the clinical aspects of her work and the psychological challenges of her consultees. On the basis of limited information and observation of Tyra's interactions with her and others, Marsha has formulated some hypotheses about Tyra's current functioning. She never challenges or raises these hypotheses with Tyra, but she uses the understanding formulated from the information to adapt and enhance her interactions. Because Patricia is also insightful and psychologically savvy, Marsha helps her to compose a picture that allows Patricia to be more empathic and therefore more successful with Tyra. The consultant's goal in discussing another is always toward increased empathy and sensitivity for each other and more successful communication and negotiation.

The consultant never reveals information about any individual that isn't already shared with others. In this case, the information comes indirectly and is only used toward the goal of greater understanding—Patricia and Rosie already have the information. Rosie's motivation for sharing may need to be considered by the consultant and addressed, but Marsha's use of that information is currently targeted toward understanding Tyra and improving the relationships with her and between Tyra and her colleagues. Because Patricia has already revealed similar history to Tyra's, Marsha rightly guesses that Patricia might be empathic to Tyra's struggles. Trying to create a different outcome for Tyra rather than the quick exits from past jobs in the face of staff conflict, Marsha attempts to prepare Patricia for possible reactions from Tyra and to plan responses that might be in tune with Tyra's needs and yet interrupt her usual routine.

However, the meetings were not without problems. As they progressed, Marsha became more and more clear that her efforts to mollify Tyra were not enough. Ironically, Tyra was desperately trying to gain Bob's acceptance, but her behavior rendered that nearly impossible in spite of Marsha's attempts to facilitate opportunities. Instead, Tyra seemed unremitting in her efforts to antagonize Bob.

Bob had finally responded to Tyra's incessant complaints and had planned and implemented a more engaging activity rather than his usual spur of the moment diversions. Usually, he didn't have to work that hard because his strong presence and the fact that he was male excited the children (for whom this was a novel experience) and kept them engaged. The toddlers failed to notice the lack of curriculum planning. Marsha was impressed with his thoughtfulness as well as his responsiveness to Tyra. Tyra was not as impressed—he had used supplies that she had put aside for an activity. Immediately, she loudly outlined his incompetence in front of the children. Bob told her to shut up. They argued until a colleague reminded them of the children who all along had been listening while being readied for nap by the lone aide. Two parents picking up their children were also privy to the fireworks.

By the time Marsha arrived, the place was buzzing. As she passed through the yard, Leticia told her to watch out. When she entered Patricia's office, she knew she'd find a hornet's nest. Tyra was already there, droning to Patricia, who called for Marsha to join them. Gaining Tyra's permission, Marsha sorted out the pieces. Despite her tirades about Bob's inconsiderateness and laziness, Tyra mainly felt taken for granted by Bob. She denied this interpretation, but Marsha kept it in mind and tried to pinpoint Tyra's wishes while trying to speak for Bob's experience. Finally, they decided on a meeting with

Bob to set up some ground rules for supplies and classroom practices. Wanting to empathize with Tyra, Marsha wasn't forceful, but she interjected that both Bob and the children's experience needed to be considered too.

A few days later, after some preparation with Patricia and with Bob, Marsha thought everyone might be ready to talk. Marsha struggled to create room for Bob because Tyra took over with complaints. It was strained, but the conversation seemed to be going well. They established rules for supplies and time for daily communication. Near the end, Bob again apologized for his past joke and his use of reserved supplies but also asked for Tyra's respect when she talked to him especially in front of children and parents. Marsha thought he had been pretty generous and deferential in his request but could see Tyra tighten up. She was silent as Marsha ended the meeting.

Tyra's therapist might have not challenged her as much, but Marsha as consultant needed to preserve respect for everyone's subjective experience. Even though Bob was much more able to tolerate the conflict, Marsha had to be aware of her relationship to him and attempt to insert his perspective in Tyra's view when possible. Although with Tyra this was nearly impossible, she had to hold the idea that Bob had a different subjective experience from Tyra's and value both. It is most important that, as a consultant, Marsha represents the children, giving voice to their experience so that it is not drowned out by the adults' conflict.

As Marsha and Patricia went back to the office and Bob went home, Tyra flew back to her classroom and began ripping children's projects off the wall. Luckily, the children were in the yard being supervised by others. It wasn't long before Leticia had alerted the office of the commotion. Patricia had had enough and threatened to fire Tyra. Marsha acknowledged the exasperation and reminded her how good Tyra could usually be with the children. She wondered if Bob's words had inadvertently shamed Tyra when she so desperately wanted to be taken care of and receive approval from this father figure. Really, Tyra appreciated the same things about him that the children did. Marsha also noted how many times Tyra had had to leave other jobs for similar reasons. Without their help she would continue to repeat this. Patricia was reminded about her own challenges with authority figures so she asked for Marsha's help. (After leaving the center, Marsha thought about the triggering conversation that she thought had been relatively benign. Bob's attempt to preserve his dignity and set some respectful boundaries had felt like criticism to Tyra. The fact that Marsha hadn't stopped him and had spoken about the effect on children compounded Tyra's embarrassment. Tyra felt betrayed by Marsha, this woman who had previously seemed to understand her and to offer support. Tyra's lifetime feelings of persecution led her to perceive all possible slights as attacks that called for retaliation. Her only power was her success as a teacher so she needed to obliterate the evidence of her teaching prowess to punish the adults who had failed to appreciate her gifts.)

Tyra came to the office threatening to quit unless Patricia handled Bob. Patricia soothed Tyra, noting her mood and frustration and expressing her own sadness if this talented teacher were to leave. With Tyra's ego tentatively buttressed, Patricia also reminded her about whose work she had removed: the children's. Tyra argued that the walls would be bare without her efforts. Although they could all agree that this was likely true, Marsha wondered if sometimes Tyra criticized or even physically moved Bob's projects with the children to less conspicuous places because they didn't meet her standards. Tyra grudgingly agreed. Marsha clarified, "It must have been so hard to hear criticism from Bob when you have tried so hard in the classroom and no one seems to see how hard you've been working." Tyra reengaged and Patricia easily followed. She reminded Tyra that just because Tyra is not privy to the conversations between her and Bob doesn't mean that she wasn't addressing Bob's performance. This seemed to mollify Tyra because she likely assumed that the reprimands for Bob were greater than they actually were. Patricia reminded her that just as this conversation would remain private so would Patricia's discussions with Bob. They all agreed, however, that Tyra might need to take some vacation time to recover. With Tyra, Marsha rehung the art projects and admired the children's and Tyra's work.

Because Marsha had already helped Patricia consider Tyra's personal challenges, Patricia was more prepared to respond sensitively to Tyra. Patricia is able to imbue her supervisory responsibilities with enough empathy to engage Tyra. This attention to the emotional experience of the staff members facilitates better communication and interrupts Tyra's usual repertoire for conflict. Rather than being fired or leaving angrily, Tyra is offered another possibility that has emerged because the consultant has helped all to consider theirs and others' intentions and the obstacles, often intrapsychic, interfering with those goals.

> Two weeks later, Tyra returns rejuvenated. Marsha and Patricia had passed the test. In the face of conflict and rage, they managed to maintain the ideas that everyone deserved respect, that the children's needs were primary, and that expectations for behavior applied to all. They had set firm boundaries, allowed her to test them, and had not rejected or shamed her. Tyra had begun to settle down and to repair her ego while Marsha prepared Bob for her return. To his surprise, Marsha explained how much those who are critical often need approval and feared rejection without revealing Tyra's particular struggles. Understanding her critical outbursts, Bob became more patient.

Without talking specifically about Tyra's history or even their interactions, Marsha offers an alternative explanation for her behavior. The consultant is always trying to broaden and shift the way that each member views themselves and others. Bob may be able to respond more empathically because he will not need to personalize Tyra's actions.

Bridging the Gap Between Adult and Child Focus

The devaluation of the profession and the difficulties in staff relationships eventually, if not immediately, affect the children. The inability to appreciate one's own and each other's feelings often results in a dismissal of or blindness to the children's experience. Eventually, providers doubt their efficacy as teachers and fail to recognize the powerful position that they hold in the lives of children. This can be a downward spiral because as people fail to see themselves as agents of change, they lose the possibility of creating shifts to improve the care and well-being of children. Tailoring responses to individual children begins to feel cumbersome, and the needs of many are even more burdensome. Relationships may come to be seen as problematic rather than pleasurable, including parent–child relationships.

The consultant addresses this problem at several levels. As discussed earlier, she works on the health of staff relationships. She also calls attention to the ways in which the children respond to caregivers. In earlier chapters, when Leo frustrated the preschool staff, the consultant highlighted times when they were successful with him and showed them how he looked to them for approval. She addressed the providers' despair about their ineffectiveness by challenging their misperceptions, and she underscored their importance.

When the implicit connection between staff actions and a child's experience seems either too threatening or impossible to consider, the consultant holds this ideal for the group. She supports and praises staff members' successes and encourages endeavors that might have the goal of improving the children's experience. For instance, Sally had recently fired her first pottery piece (a beautiful bowl). She had been talking enthusiastically about her accomplishment with her coworkers and the consultant who had voiced interest. The moment was noteworthy because it was one of the rare times that Sally actually seemed excited about something. She was usually sullen and removed from her colleagues and the children. Her interactions with the children were most often limited to scolding and custodial supervision. With the consultant's encouragement, Sally brought her bowl in to share with her coworkers who, led by the consultant, all responded with praise, enlivening Sally. The consultant built on this excitement, "Sally, your work is so impressive, I'm sure that the children would love to work with clay too." At first Sally resisted until the consultant scaled down the project, "Perhaps, you could show them your work during circle time and then put out clay at the activity table. I think they would really love it, I can see how happy your work has made you." The consultant's enthusiasm eventually rubbed off, and, for the first time, Sally was excited about her interactions with the children. The attention to the children was only possible because the consultant had paid attention to Sally.

When possible, the consultant reconnects these successes to the impact that they have on the children. When Sally introduced clay to the children, they took to it with gusto. The tactile experience and the tangible product captured them thoroughly. The consultant had several goals. She underscored the children's enthusiasm, to which Sally had become inured. She made the connection between Sally's feelings of excitement and the children's engaged efforts, in an attempt to connect one to the other. Because Sally and others have lost confidence and a sense of value in their work, they fail to see the connection between the children's interests and their own and between the children's growth and change and their efforts. The consultation can rebuild this connection. Increases in the caregivers' self-efficacy and competence were evidenced in an evaluation of child-care centers that received consultation for more than a year (Alkon, Ramler, & Mac Lennan, 2003).

Case Example, Continued

We return to Bread and Jam Child Care after some of the difficulties had been resolved. Excitement in an activity changed the culture of the toddler room, but the consultant needed to make the connection between the staff's actions and the children's responsiveness.

> Although Marsha had not observed the toddler room in the beginning of the year, she remembered seeing clusters of crying children attached to one of the aides every time she passed through the yard in the first few months. She had wondered about this with Patricia, but all seemed to believe that this was how children entered any early childhood program. If you just ignored the crying long enough, it would go away. They had never had a new charge cry for more than 2 months, in their minds proving them right.

The ability to disconnect and thereby summarily dismiss children's distress when separated from their parents for the first time gives perspective on the defenses providers erect to keep from feeling or at least feeling more than they can manage. We have argued that this lack of responsiveness is accounted for by the dearth of these experiences for adults, past or present. Even when teachers' histories are benign or better, the current societal treatment of child-care professionals and the associated functioning of the adult relationships can close adults off to their own and then to the children's emotional experience.

In April, when the school first began considering which toddlers would transfer to the preschool class and who was leaving for kindergarten, Marsha decided to address the beginning of the year transition especially for new toddlers. Marsha was persistent. She planned meetings on the subject with Patricia, offered trainings, encouraged planning meetings and specific activities, and spoke for the children's experience. Although all seemed to acknowledge the importance of transitions, they didn't believe that the crying could be curtailed. August, September, and October passed with wailing children clustered around the one nurturing aide. Marsha watched helplessly and vowed that the following year would be better.

Throughout the year, Marsha took every opportunity to underscore the importance of transitions—large and small. When April came again, she tried to turn attention to preparing for the arrival of new toddlers, stressing the benefits to the staff if children entered more easily. Again, staff seemed interested but not particularly enthusiastic, and more pressing concerns arose. Marsha looked for openings.

In the meantime, Patricia had been writing grants and had received one to enhance the art curriculum. Tyra had convinced her to buy a digital camera for documentation. Soon, Tyra was creating interactive projects with the children—Marsha was impressed and shared that with Tyra. Bob was also impressed and perhaps a little jealous. He wanted to learn how to use it.

Tyra enjoyed the power this dynamic conferred. This made Marsha nervous, but Bob seemed able to tolerate it. Soon enough, he too was using the camera to take pictures of the staff and children, and Tyra was helping him to modify and print them. Both were proudly bringing their latest portraits to the group meetings. Marsha wondered if they might use this new skill at the beginning of the year because children love to see pictures of themselves and their family. Displaying staff pictures might familiarize parents with their children's providers, allaying apprehension about the strangers with whom they were leaving their precious babies. Marsha reminded them about last year.

Tyra and Bob quickly expanded these ideas. By the time the new school year arrived, there were labeled portraits of the staff as well as the regular substitutes greeting the families as they arrived. Impromptu shots were taken of each family on the day they began and were placed in their child's cubby with a copy for home. Near the sign-in sheet, Bob had created a rotating presentation of the week's activities. Parents began to stop and chat with the morning and afternoon staff and also began to donate printer paper so that they could have copies for home.

A video camera extended the outreach. The growing success through the summer of pictures had also encouraged Bob to bring in his video camera. By September's Open House, he had a full-length video of the children's experience at school. The parents were fascinated. Tyra supplemented the presentation by giving tours of the different activity centers in the room—demonstrating how each was used, how each provided a basis for learning, and how the children approached the areas. By the end of the evening, Bob had also recorded each parent in the area of their choosing, talking about what they liked about it and what they thought their child might enjoy. Later, Bob would use this video to soothe children who missed their parents. Even Tyra was impressed and a year and a half after their blow-up was beginning to appreciate Bob's contribution.

At the next staff meeting, Marsha was electrified by all of their excitement over the beginning of the year. All agreed that the parents really enjoyed the parent meeting, it was their best turnout and greatest involvement—some parents even wanted to volunteer in the classroom—a first for this usually uninvolved parent community. Marsha thought to her self, "I better underline these transition successes," and wondered what staff made of this and the very few tears shed this year. Most of the children had become comfortable so quickly that it felt like the beginning of November rather than mid-September.

Instead of connecting it to their recent efforts as Marsha expected, the staff attributed the diminished distress to an especially easy group of kids. They reported that they were mostly girls. "Wasn't it just as often girls whose sobbing persisted last year?" she questioned. They had to admit that it was but had a difficult time naming other reasons. When Marsha connected the children's and parent's behavior to the teacher's actions and preparations, it was uniformly rejected to Marsha's consternation.

In supervision, Marsha expressed surprise and frustration with the lack of staff enthusiasm for her interpretation of the classroom's recent turnaround. She was afraid that the lack of understanding would mean that as the passion for the digital camera waned so would the activities supporting transition. "What stopped them from considering their involvement?" wondered her supervisor. Marsha no longer resisted this line of questioning, she recognized the prompting as encouragement to reflect—the same thing she had learned to do with the providers. As they considered together the impediments, Marsha remembered how much the staff needed approval from her and Patricia. The societal devaluing of their roles had subverted their sense of efficacy. They couldn't see themselves or their actions as the agents of positive change in the children. How could they appreciate the power of their transition efforts when they had abandoned the premise that had brought them to the field—that caregiver efforts could help children?

With her supervisor's help, Marsha found the language to convey this loss, "I was thinking about our discussion last week and how you explained the beginning of the year's ease to factors outside your control. It made me sad to think how little you give credit to yourselves." Continuing, she drew clear connections between their actions over the time she had been there and the observable shifts in the classroom and the children. Not completely convinced, they did smile shyly at the thought of their powerful presence. Despite her efforts, the group would remain cautious about accepting a sense of control. The weight of the realization was daunting. If they could be positive influences, they had to consider that the opposite might be equally possible. It was sometimes easier to be unaware, but Marsha would keep finding opportunities to confirm their efforts and question their willingness to abdicate their importance.

When providers find the right rhythm with a particularly challenging child, that new-found skill and confidence often generalizes to greater responsiveness to others. A small shift will ripple through the whole system. In the previous section, attention to adult relationships, and to Tyra's in particular, resulted in better services for children. Their transition eased, the children felt more secure, and in turn the parents became more invested in the program and in their role as parents.

These ripples are not limited to the provider–child relationships or even the staff–parent relationships. A parallel process also flows to and through the consultation relationship. The good feelings engendered in the preschool room about the consultant had allowed the consultant access to the toddler room. Just as the teachers have to accept that along with the possible positive effects of their actions on the children come times of temporary struggle, the consultant must also watch for the ways in which her actions may have negative consequences no matter how inadvertent.

During the same time period that the consultant, Marsha, was addressing the needs of the toddler room, she continued to meet with the staff of the preschool room. The head teacher Stacey and her assistants Harold and Leticia had all become quite comfortable with Marsha. Marsha began to take the ease of this relationship for granted. As things were going well with this team, she had been focusing most of her energy and enthusiasm on the toddler room. We return to Bread and Jam Child Care's preschool room just as Marsha's involvement with Tyra and Bob was being fully noticed by the preschool staff.

> By this time, Marsha had already begun to address parent relationships with the preschool staff, but the excitement of the digital pictures and communication spread like a cold among preschool children. Sandra, Leticia, and Harold became a little jealous of the focus placed on the toddler room's success with parents. They wanted their own digital camera. They talked about wanting more involvement with parents and about the newfangled technology to do it. They wanted a digital camera and were not enamored of sharing it with Tyra. Eventually, Patricia found funds, and the object of everyone's desire was purchased for the preschool. Rarely was it used.

The urgency for more immediate parent involvement is, like a sudden shift in a child's behavior, an indicator that the staff is responding to change in the environment. Although due partially to movement in the toddler room and the wish for similar supplies, the consultant registers possible deeper meanings. The preschool staff's clamoring for "more involvement" and their insistence on "not sharing" may in fact be related to their relationship with her.

> Marsha's obvious enthusiasm for the shift in the toddler classroom had its own consequences. Leticia and Stacey began to remind Marsha and Patricia of their own successes in the classroom. Now 2 years later, they still spoke about Leo and how well he was doing in first grade. Leticia saw his mother in the community regularly and received updates, which she shared proudly. In fact, at times, Marsha used that first-year experience to remind them of the ups and downs of progress when the team was particularly discouraged by a challenging or regressing child or parent. Reminders of Leo's achievement and theirs with him always lifted their spirits.

It was only in supervision that she realized that they were jealous of Marsha's interest in Bob and Tyra's triumph. They were reminding Marsha of their own victories more often because they missed being the center of Marsha's attention. The first year of her arrival, they had received Marsha's focus and basked in the glory of her accolades and patience. They were seen, understood, and appreciated. Marsha, who had been new to consulting, had failed to see the conferred power of her role. Two-and-a-half years later, she was facing the effects of that power and of her failure to acknowledge it.

Marsha had begun to take for granted the shifts in the preschool teacher's abilities and their classroom's functioning. They noticed that she talked to them like colleagues and enjoyed the camaraderie, but they missed the praise—an experience in short supply in this traditionally undervalued field.

In supervision, Marsha stopped to consider the progress that they had made. Along the way, she, like the toddler staff, had to be reminded of her contribution and participation in the accomplishments. Back in the preschool's weekly meetings, she said, "I've been thinking about our work together and how much has happened. We work so easily together and things flow so smoothly, I forget to recognize how much effort you've expended in making a great class." Each of the members smiled in appreciation. Together they revisited their success.

Adults need praise just as children do. When they are struggling with new endeavors, reminders of prior successful battles can increase frustration tolerance. These needs arise again as new struggles arise.

As much as the work might feel circumscribed, the consultant's actions will be considered throughout the center. The consultant's ability to accept her limitations and hear them from the participants will go along way toward fostering direct communication among child-care providers and with parents. This modeling becomes particularly useful for teachers in the parallel teacher–parent relationship.

Parent–Staff Relationships

Sometimes the lack of respect for the profession and for each other can leak to the relationships with parents. Parents and staff see each other for brief moments and yet share the incredible task of raising children. As among teachers, child-rearing views between parents and staff can vary greatly. The differences are exacerbated when they are unidentified but the children act out the discrepancy. Recrimination and blaming become the only mode of communication for adults.

Although we address teacher–parent relationships more fully in subsequent chapters, the tenets in this chapter are particularly useful. Whenever possible, the consultant attempts to foster direct communication among the teachers and parents. She can do so by preventively anticipating parents' needs and frustrations. Planning the inclusion of parents can preempt later difficulties. Always, she is increasing the level of understanding between the adults. She wants each to understand the stresses of the others' challenges while she offers support for theirs. Whenever possible, she asks them to imagine what the other feels. When they are unable to do so because of anger or ignorance, she translates the perspectives in language and examples that will be most salient to the listener. Although the consultant wishes for direct communication between parent and teacher, she accepts that sometimes the contentiousness has become too fevered and she must serve as the bridge between the two.

When members of a child-care team feel more able to negotiate with each other, they bring this competency, and perhaps this openness, to their relationships with parents. In Bread and Jam's toddler room and earlier in the preschool room, as the staff became more able to understand each other and the children, they began to bring this understanding to the parents. The consultant, Marsha, assisted this process by helping the teachers see the parents' perspectives. Often the consultant stops and asks providers to consider their own experiences in similar situations before she asks them to offer empathy to the parents.

In the previous chapter, we left Bread and Jam Child Care while the preschool staff was instituting a policy to greet all parents to ease the morning transition for the children and to involve parents. Although this worked immediately for some parents, others were less responsive. Leticia, a great-grandmother, struggled with what she perceived as a lack of respect from parents who kept their heads down and hurried out of the classroom. When Leticia became angry, the consultant spent time with her considering the meaning of respect in her life. As a great-grandmother, she felt she deserved deference from these young parents. The conversation went something like this:

> Marsha wondered how Leticia had taught her own children to greet adults. Leticia summed it up simply, "They knew better than to disrespect an adult." Leticia had developed a fondness for Marsha so she could get away with chuckling, "I bet they did." Marsha then shared with them how her own mother would whisper in her ear before meeting new people, "Remember to say hello and shake their hand." "In fact, she did it the last time I visited her," she laughed, as did the group. Stacy, Patricia, and Leticia began to share their own experiences of being taught and teaching manners. Harold shared that although he had prepared his son for social interactions, no one had done it for him. It took him a long time to figure out how to move in the world. Marsha wondered if perhaps some of the parents were struggling like he had. To understand this phenomenon, the group added information about the parents that they knew from the community. Marsha added additional interpretations, "Perhaps, they're also shy." Leticia doubted this, but Marsha teased, "You're pretty tough, Leticia. As you said, you could be their grandmother—that's kind of intimidating—because of course you know more than they do about bringing up children." Leticia liked this. But it also reminded all of them what it meant to be young parents.

> Marsha wondered what it was like for these parents whose children seemed to love coming here. These parents worked all day, leaving their children with someone else to raise—someone who might do it better. Stacey was suddenly moved by how hard it was for the parents. As they began to talk about those challenges and how to help them, Leticia added that she could make more conversation with the parents in the morning. All agreed to do this.

The consultant was able to pursue this line of questioning because she had consistently offered a nonjudgmental ear. When teachers shared personal information, they felt safe and protected. They also knew that the consultant used this information to gain better understanding, not for recriminations. The consultant's own experiences demonstrated how information from one's own life can be used to better understand that of others. Empathy is learned both by receiving it consistently and through instruction— "How would you feel if…" The consultant did both just as the teachers did with the children in their care.

> Soon there was a shift in the morning routine. Parents were lingering in the classroom to complain about their morning, to ask questions, to share weekend activities, and to disclose other intimacies. Leticia gathered information and shared it with the other teachers because she loved to gossip. Unfortunately, this also meant that she shared family secrets with any parents who were curious. Marsha helped them to consider the parents' experience, "I'm sure that they enjoy the details, but I wonder if they think twice about sharing their own information with you." With a big extended family, Leticia could relate to the misunderstandings of too many people telling a story. Not completely successful in maintaining boundaries, she was able to curtail most of her inappropriate disclosures.

The consultant can speak for the parents' experience, but she can also help teachers develop and voice their own understanding of the parents. Although the first is often more accurate (because the consultant as an outsider can remain more objective), the latter is usually more effective in engendering empathy for parents. When a consultant has properly prepared a child-care team by listening intently with the wish to understand, the child-care team is usually more able to offer this to parents as well as to the children. The consultant can also use her knowledge of the teachers to make greater and more poignant connections between their and the parents' experience. She can model this as Marsha did by sparingly offering her own experiences.

As the teacher–parent relationships become closer and comfortable, more information is shared. Confidentiality and privacy need to be discussed directly as providers become privy to family news.

Summary

Child care is a highly interpersonal field. The needs of children are constant and require emotional presence. Add to this logistics: shared space and duties, demanding constant negotiation and flexibility. The demands of raising children together challenge most parent couples. When you assemble a staff who have not chosen each other and may have very different ideas and customs regarding children and child rearing, those difficulties expand exponentially.

Furthermore, the general devaluation of child care expressed most particularly in pay but also in general respect for the child-care profession takes its toll on the self-worth of staff. Because this process is so global and not easily labeled, teachers may lash out at each other. In addition, the child-care profession attracts those who want to work with children but may have less acumen and interest in collaborating with adults.

While addressing particulars about a program's functioning, the consultant must also repair and build the relationships among the staff. The health of these relationships directly affects the well-being of the children in their care. The consultant involves the director, first gaining her trust and establishing the importance of considering the subjective experience of her staff. Because directors have often been promoted from the ranks, they sometimes lack the supervisory skills necessary for their roles. The consultant may attempt to help her to become more effective, usually by focusing on her relationships with her supervisees.

In the larger staff group, the consultant works toward having individuals express themselves appropriately and speak directly to each other. Occasionally, direct interactions are too threatening so that the consultant might be the conduit for staff members' communications in the beginning. This raises issues of confidentiality and privacy and borders the arena of therapy. Although the consultant is always concerned about confidentiality for the children and staff, her primary goal is helping the group function better. To this end, she asserts the usefulness of sharing information and assists in encouraging personal disclosure that is pertinent to programmatic practices and staff's ways of viewing and relating to one another. As always, the consultant understands that in order for individuals to appreciate the subjective experience of their peers, they must feel heard and understood themselves. Sometimes, the consultant provides this space before encouraging direct interaction. In the process, she helps to translate the perspective and concerns of each member to maximize the potential for understanding among the group.

When staff have repaired and fostered their own relationships, they will also be more open to responding to and thinking about parents. The consultant brings the same concepts to the consideration of these relationships, always helping one person understand the perspective and experience of another. When possible, she helps staff institute systemic changes to be more inclusive of parents.

References

Alkon, A., Ramler, M., & MacLennan, K. (2003). Evaluation of mental health consultation in child care centers. *Early Childhood Education Journal, 31* (2), 91–99.

James Bowman Associates & Kagan, F. L. (2003). *Evaluation report on mental health consultation to child-care centers.* San Francisco: Jewish Family and Children's Services. Retrieved February 2005 from http://www.jfcs.org/search/default.aspx?term=Evaluation+mental+health+consultation

Pawl, J. H., & Johnston, K. (1991, August 12). *Daycare Consultants Program final reports to the Stuart Foundation: Process evaluation report.* San Francisco.

Chapter 6

Beginning Case Consultation: Gaining Entry and Setting the Tone

In this chapter, our voyage into consultation around a specific child starts—case consultation. The journey can be complicated, so we will follow the phases and activities over this and several subsequent chapters. Our travels along the consultative course are illustrated by examining one child's experience in more depth. The child, Justin, and the consultative activities that take place around him and on his behalf, guide us through the meandering channels of case consultation. Case consultation follows the same principles and stance already articulated in the process of program consultation. To whom the principles are applied expands to include the child's family.

From the moment a request is made, case consultation considers the nature of the request, the individuals asking for help, and the context out of which it arises. Case and program consultation intersect as both the characteristics of the child-care program as well as the description of the child offer useful information. The consultant's flexibility in tacking back and forth between a child and the child-care context is the first leg of the consultative trip.

Introducing the provider's wish for consultation, securing parental permission, and involving the child's family in the process are equally important activities of the initial phase. Once agreement is reached among providers, parents, and the consultant, the journey of understanding the child's behavior begins.

Linking Case and Program Consultation

Whether the request to focus on a particular child begins the consultation relationship or it emerges from an ongoing consultation that has focused on programmatic issues or other children, the consultant always moves between case and program content. The consultant's stance and the principles informing practice are identical. She applies them in new and varied contexts. The child's family is incorporated into the sphere of adults who the consultant engages and whose perspective of the child the consultant takes into account. The child and the meaning of his behavior is, obviously, the content discussed in case consultation conversations.

In previous chapters, the consultant's "way of being" and the principles guiding consultation were applied to general programmatic issues. The contribution that consultation can make in addressing interstaff difficulties and program practices was highlighted. Although a child, Leo appeared regularly, the broader issues effecting overall quality were purposefully put to the forefront. These broader content conversations are often interwoven with and are an outgrowth of consultation around a specific child. Leo served as the catalyst for the staff and consultant's expansion into diverse but related program issues, which impacted the overall quality of care. Reciprocally, all the areas addressed in program consultation affected Leo. In this section of the book, a shifted vantage point brings the child into bold relief. But before turning our lens totally, we want to look at the ebb and flow between case and program consultation as a consultant is required to move fluidly between the two. Looking at this intersection is also important because the consultant must consider the child-care context even as she begins case consultation.

Child-care providers often seek mental health consultation for the first time when they are especially worried, alarmed, or perplexed by the behavior of a particular child. Providers likely equate mental health services exclusively with direct, individual intervention. Therefore, they may feel that the usefulness of mental health consultation is limited to particularly acute situations involving a specific child. Traditionally, mental health professionals enter the child-care picture, if at all, when concerns about an individual child seem serious enough to indicate their involvement.

Reasons for Focus on Child

Our experience has taught us that case consultation is asked for initially even when more comprehensive mental health consultation is available. The reasons that requests for case consultation precede those for program consultation are myriad. Feelings of desperation provoked by the pain of a child about whom providers care deeply may lead them to seek help when they would not otherwise feel the need. Alternately, a child might act as the "identified patient," representing and responding to broader systemic problems.

Feels safer

Beginning with case consultation circumvents acknowledging or directly asking for assistance in programmatic problems. Exposing systemic difficulties to an outsider who is not yet known or trusted by the adults in the program can feel more threatening than talking about a child. While providers may be worried, they usually do not feel they are the cause of a child's difficulties. However, they may feel responsible for programmatic shortcomings.

Creates openings for addressing programmatic challenges

Case consultation, while benefiting an individual child, can simultaneously create openings for the consultant's expanded involvement in program consultation. Establishing a relationship with caregivers in which their subjective experience of a child is appreciated goes far toward developing trust between consultant and consultees. When caregivers discover the usefulness of understanding a child's needs as well as appreciate the programmatic influences on one child's behavior and then his peers, they often request program consultation. Because case consultation necessarily seeks to understand systemic issues, caregivers are already prepared for programmatic discussions.

Understanding the Provider–Child Relationship

The factors contributing to a child's developmental and behavioral difficulties may predate and exceed their involvement in child care. Although not necessarily causative, the provider–child relationship is central to effecting any positive change in the child. This relationship cannot be meaningfully considered or addressed separate from the many systems in which it exists and unfolds. In case, as in program consultation, the consultant attempts to understand as much as possible about the program's philosophy and daily routines as well as about interstaff and parent–staff relationships. The consultant develops an understanding of each provider's role expectations, emotional capacities, and beliefs about development as these are inevitably expressed in the provider's attitude toward and relationship with all children.

Flexible Shifts in Attention

Flexibility is a hallmark of the consultative approach. (a) As consultation occurs outside an office, the traditional trappings that signal the rules and boundaries of a treatment relationship are missing. The consultant cannot rely on the 50-minute hour or her office door to establish beginnings and endings. She must carry the parameters of her position with her as she moves within a setting over which she has little say and even less control. (b) She must get to know and equally attend to the requests and needs of children, parents, providers, and directors while juggling the meaning her involvement has with any one of them to the others. (c) Finally, and most specifically relevant to our discussion of case consultation, the consultant nimbly shifts attention between individual children and the environment. To assist a child, she must understand and address the relationships in which he lives while attending to the program's ability and readiness to address his needs. As we explore case consultation in depth, we are reminded of the consultant's continual need to reposition herself.

Case Example

In this chapter, we meet the staff of the Good Days Child Care Center as they request consultation around Justin. Because the consultant is involved at many levels with all of the adults in Justin's life, we follow this case through this and all subsequent chapters. As the first scenes are described, we ask you to pay particular attention to the ways in which the consultant incorporates and attends to a variety of issues and perspectives within the child-care community and between the child-care providers and this child's guardian.

The staff of Good Days Child Care Center was becoming increasingly concerned about Justin, a 2½ year-old boy who had been at the center for just 3 months. Justin was initially quite withdrawn and quiet, rarely expressing preference for, or pleasure in, any of the day's happenings. Staff often overlooked his meek bids for interaction or assistance until he began lashing out at peers who approached him during play or sat close to him at snack or circle time. Transitions were becoming problematic. When outside time was announced, Justin held tight to whatever object had been occupying his attention, refusing to relinquish it for the trip to a nearby park. Once he was cajoled or carried to the playground, he could momentarily settle himself with sand or wheel toys. The route back to the center was harrowing as Justin routinely planted himself in the busy intersection between the play yard and the center. Often exhausted after this journey, the providers began to dread Justin's post-lunch transition to naptime. Justin alternately bolted from his cot or wound himself in a web of his bedding, all the while shrieking loudly enough to keep most of the other children awake.

The consultant, who had a 3-year relationship with the center, had heard snippets of this description in earlier meetings. Today, Justin's increasing difficulties took center stage as she sat with the program's recently reconfigured staff. Sue, the lead teacher, had been working in this program for nearly 10 years. She was raised and still lived just down the street from the center. Her familiarity with the neighborhood was both a blessing and a hardship. She knew many of the parents whose children attended the program as they too had remained in this impoverished, deteriorating, and often crime-riddled area. Consequently, Sue was widely respected and trusted by the families of her child-care charges. However, the blurring of personal and professional identities was at times confusing for both Sue and the parents. The two other providers, Latania and Tometrius, had recently been relocated to this center. They were transferred from another program under the same administration. Neither embraced the change enthusiastically as they felt they had not been consulted about or given a choice in the change.

Listening to the caregivers' frustrations and concerns about Justin, the consultant first empathized with and then asked the group if they were considering consultation specifically focused on Justin. Everyone agreed that something needed to be done. This is where the agreement ended. The group sat in silence. Given their long-standing relationship, the consultant knew that Sue understood the need to obtain Justin's grandmother's permission to discuss and to observe him further. Given that Sue likely knew Justin's grandmother, her silence seemed conspicuous.

In an attempt to acknowledge Sue's experience with consultation and to promote direct communication among colleagues, the consultant asked if Sue had had an opportunity to talk with the others about the "ways we usually begin case consultation or if she wanted to now." Sue's slight shake of the head and downward glance indicated an unrevealed obstacle.

The consultant directed herself to the two new caregivers, "I know we haven't focused on a specific child since you've been here, so it probably didn't mean much when I talked about case consultation at one of our first meetings. When we want to think together about a child like Justin we always want to start by letting the parents know you want my help." Getting only mumbled grunts of understanding from the group the consultant persevered, "So are there any ideas about how it would be best to talk with Justin's grandma?" The consultant plows through the stony silence, "It seems like something is making it difficult to consider this? Is there something about speaking with grandma that's hard?"

The discussion revealed broader concerns related to interstaff difficulties and disparate ideas about parent–staff relationships. It was unanimously agreed that Sue, the veteran staff member, had the closest relationship with Mrs. Jones (Justin's grandmother) and would be the best person to introduce the wish for consultation, but Sue expressed apprehension, "Yeah I know Pauline, I mean Mrs. Jones, but I don't want to step on peoples' toes by talking to her. I am not the only one who can talk to parents." Sue sputtered in the direction of her co-teachers. Catching on, the consultant wondered if the issue at hand was only tangentially related to Justin and to acquiring consent. "So it seems less like a question of who should talk to Mrs. Jones and more about how it's been feeling between all of you. I realize we jumped right into talking about children. We haven't paid nearly as much attention to how the change has been for the three of you as you're trying to find ways of working together. I probably could have noticed sooner. I'm just recognizing you all started working together at about the same time Justin arrived. It must make it hard to sort out all of what's contributing to it feeling so difficult to support him. It seems like it might be difficult to discuss Justin until we spend some time thinking about your relationships with each other and with the parents. How would you like to proceed?" The providers tentatively acknowledged the need to sort out issues related to their respective roles, especially pertaining to their interactions with the parents of all the children in their care.

As the consultant explored this with the group, it became apparent that the new staff members were both suspicious and envious of Sue's relationships, not only with Justin's grandmother but also with all parents. They resented her and the parents who they felt had not welcomed them. In response they had withdrawn from virtually all parent contact. That left Sue feeling overburdened and resentful as she felt solely responsible for responding to all the parents.

The consultant's focus expanded, but she did not lose sight of Justin. With the providers' permission, several subsequent consultation meetings dealt with the broader issues of interstaff and parent–staff relationships. In these discussions the consultant invited each of the newer teachers to talk more about their experience of leaving a center in which they felt competent and comfortable. She emphasized the idea that change, when one has no choice, can influence one's perspective about the new experience. She posited parallels to Justin's experience of entering an unfamiliar place: the child-care center.

The consultant also elicited Sue's story as the sole staff member left holding the program's history and the neighborhood's legacy. Sue felt responsible and compensated by doing as much as she could for every family. As she spoke, Sue became more aware that her burden was self-imposed, yet she resented the disproportionate weight she carried. The consultant created and protected space for each participant's voice, remarking on how understandable their misinterpretations of each other's actions and attitudes were. Sue rushed in as the others backed off. Neither understood the reasons behind the other's actions. The intentions behind their behaviors became clear as the conversations with the consultant continued.

The consultant identified the ways in which these misinterpretations contributed to distrust and difficulty among the teachers and with the parents. The consultant linked the providers' intentions and feelings to the outcome. Sue felt increasingly unable to rely on her coworkers while they saw her relationship with the parents as a conspiracy to keep them out. Disentangling the complicated feelings the teachers had toward their jobs and one another allowed them to consider more satisfactory solutions to the dilemma that had developed with parents. Together they decided to officially welcome the new teachers at the next monthly parent meeting. Inadvertently, the newer providers had not been acknowledged or formally introduced despite their presence at two prior parent gatherings.

By wondering what they would say about themselves to the parents, the consultant helped the team to consider their roles as part of a unit working on the behalf of the children. By noticing their hard work toward developing a team and devotion to the children, the consultant established enough goodwill to have the group ponder the parents' experience. She wondered how the parents perceived the emotional distance. Beginning to envision the parents' experience, the staff empathized with the families. The providers spontaneously started to speak of ways of repairing their relationships with parents. Having helped the group set up a system of primary caregiving, the consultant wondered if a description of this practice might be one way of connecting with parents. She suggested that the parents' meeting might be the place to talk about the meaning of and reasons for having primary caregivers. She added that the staff could inform families as to which provider was their child's primary caregiver.

The consultant deliberately shifted the spotlight from Justin to the adult relationships. Had she marched merrily along with the agenda of garnering consent from Justin's guardian, she would have overlooked an opportunity to address the underlying interstaff concerns. These difficulties, if unattended to, would have undoubtedly festered and multiplied and would have interfered in the consideration of Justin's needs.

The flexible shifting of attention demonstrates an essential consultative skill. The consultant responds to shifting impediments to thinking about a child. Here, Justin receded to the background as the consultant attended to the channels of communication, moving between case-centered and programmatic consultation.

The consultant adheres to the belief that general programmatic issues influence the program's ability to think about and respond well to individual children. Classroom conundrums, at times, also contribute to a specific child's distress. While focusing on overall program concerns, the consultant watches for how these difficulties might be mirrored by the child. The consultant pursued the conversation about parent–staff and interstaff difficulties while keeping in mind that these troubles have some meaning in relation to Justin. This is not to suggest that a program's problems are the sole cause of a child's concerns, but they undoubtedly exacerbate his distress.

Being pulled in many different directions can cause the consultant to question her ability to balance everyone's agenda. Although Justin's needs tugged for the consultant's immediate response, the caregivers were equally distressed. Even inside the adult arena, the consultant felt conflicted. Knowing Sue well and feeling over-worked herself, the consultant empathized intensely with Sue's sense of burden and inflated responsibility. The consultant had to dig deeper to empathize with the two new caregivers. She had to remind herself that their reluctance to extend themselves to parents protected them from the pain of separation. They had been removed from their previous positions with no warning or consideration of their wishes. As the consultant understood their behavior toward parents as a reen-actment of their own treatment, her empathy for them increased. The consult-ant adds her own internal responses to the information she gains from her consultees. The consultant directed her remarks to the areas she felt would best assist the caregivers in better understanding one another, promoting the possi-bility of their working cooperatively on behalf of Justin and the other children.

Case Consultation—Purpose and Process

Case consultation contemplates the meaning of a child's behavior, engages all of the adults in the child's life, and attempts to adapt their responses to the child's needs. The particular child-care center, family, and child add uniquely to the pro-ceedings, but a common course can be described in general phases.

In the first phase—*receiving and responding to a request*—the consultant collects information about the child, determines the nature of the request, and the con-text for the child's situation. To this end, she includes the parents, inquires about the providers' and parents' perceptions of the child, and learns about the child-care milieu including the parent–provider relationship.

In the next phase, *the co-construction of meaning*, the information is sifted through, expanded upon, and integrated. Information is obtained from providers and parents as well as through the consultant's observation. The consultant, together with the child's parents and providers, develops mutually agreed-upon hypotheses for understanding the child's development and the meaning expressed through behavior. In the final phase—*responsive action*—understanding is translated into intervention. These phases overlap and interact, but are separated here for ease of explication.

Request for Case Consultation

Case consultation is most often requested by child-care providers. A request may come in the form of a phone intake with a director or staff member who has not previously received consultation but whose worries about a child in her care provoke a call. Alternately, being asked to consider a little one whose behavior is puzzling can occur in the context of an ongoing consultative relationship in which several children and many program issues have been attended to over time. Occasionally, in programs where the consultant's presence is regular and her involvement longstanding, parents will request case consultation. Regardless of who does the asking, both parent's and provider's involvement is essential from the beginning.

When the child-care providers' questions or concerns about a child prompt the request, the consultant asks about the consultees' experience of and response to the child (see chapter 2, Initiating Consultation). The consultant conveys interest in hearing a general description of the child and the providers' concerns. The consultant also asks about and empathizes with the caregivers' experience of worry, wondering, frustration, or uncertainty. However, she discourages the disclosure of identifying information. Specific information about the child is shared with the consultant only with the parents' knowledge and consent.

Asserting Parental Centrality

While listening to caregiver's concerns or quandaries about a child, the consultant is poised to introduce the idea that parents have an essential place in the process. If providers do not spontaneously include the parents' view in describing a child's situation, the consultant asserts her idea of its importance. She may do so through simple inquiries such as, "Do Josiah's parents share your concern?" or "Has Joanna's mom been able to offer ideas about her behavior that help you make sense of what's going on for her?" The consultant poses these questions with a dual purpose in mind. Ascertaining the parent's view, whether directly or from the providers, assists the consultant in understanding a child's behavior. The consultant also cultivates the notion that the parents will need to be informants and allies in the effort to understand and assist their child.

The providers' responses offer insight into the tenor of the parent–provider relationship, and the consultant positions herself accordingly. Hearing that the adults in a child's life are unified in their concern, the consultant will likely be able to capitalize on the already established spirit of cooperation. She can anticipate that her introduction to the parents will be welcomed. Conversely, her questions may expose disagreement between parents and providers about the existence of, or cause of, the child's distress in child care. Repairing the fractured parent–provider relationship becomes the first priority. Between these two poles, other possibilities exist. Sometimes little information about how a child is faring has been exchanged between parents and providers. A nonexistent or distant provider–parent relationship precludes dialogue. Even within an established relationship, a provider may curtail communication with a parent when she is unsure about the accuracy of her assessment or apprehensive about a parent's reply. Because she lacks confidence in her opinion about the child, the provider may hope that the consultant's "expert status" will confer validity to the parents. Also, a provider may want to avoid unnecessarily upsetting or alarming the parents.

While holding steadfast to the importance of parent participation, the consultant responds to a provider's hesitancy. Child-care providers must be convinced that parent involvement is crucial, not simply so consultation can proceed but, more importantly, for their eventual efficacy with a child. The reasons for parental permission and involvement may seem obvious but at times are perceived by providers as an impediment to immediately receiving the assistance they desire.

Gaining Parental Permission

Because the consultant waits for parental permission to become involved, the providers usually introduce consultation to parents. To ensure the best introduction of her services, the consultant prepares the provider. The provider must be comfortable conveying what consultation is and why it is wanted. So together they think about the least threatening and most congenial way to introduce the services to the family. The particulars of the invitation are fashioned from information provided by the teachers. If requested, the consultant clarifies or expands upon the provider's proposed description of who the consultant is and how she might be involved.

Providing general ways of describing mental health consultation is especially useful to child-care staff who have not previously participated in case consultation. The consultant suggests that parents are likely to respond best to an offer that honors their role and identifies the child-care providers' wish to help their child, without alarming or indicting the parents. Initial focus is placed on the consultant's role in helping the providers to understand and respond better to the child. To this end, the consultant thinks with the provider about an introduction such as, "Ms. Garcia, we've been talking for a while now about our wish to help Jose feel comfortable here at our school. I know you, more than anyone, want him to feel secure and safe here. We've all been a bit stumped lately by his continued distress, but I had an idea. Our program has access to a consultant. We would like to see if she could help us better understand how to help Jose feel more settled in our school. Of course we need your permission to have her work with us. I imagine you want time to think it over, maybe to talk to your husband? Also, the consultant, her name is Graziella, would welcome talking with you. You may have questions about who she is and what she would be doing with us and for your family that would be best discussed directly with her. You could get a sense of her and see if she seems like someone you would want to have thinking with all of us about Jose."

Wishing to leap over the sometimes difficult process of procuring permission, providers at times ask consultants to "take a peek" at a child about whom they are concerned. Seduced by a sense of her own power or a provider's desperation, a consultant observes a child or dives directly into an in-depth discussion before parents are privy to her presence. The consultant must remind herself and the providers of why these actions are ill-advised. Proceeding without parents' knowledge demonstrates a lack of respect for their position. Additionally, parents are not likely to trust the expressed sentiment that their participation is vital if they are invited to join an effort that is already underway.

Providers can be swayed slightly by considering the adverse effects of excluding parents. The consultant explains that parents will likely feel tricked and therefore less likely to cooperate in an endeavor, which they are asked to join after the fact.

Speaking with parents about the wish for the consultant's help can be awkward if it is not imbedded in an already established relationship based on the staff and parents' continuous communication about the child's experience in the program. Even when communication has occurred, identification of a child's having difficulties in the program can cause a fissure in the relationship, which contributes to a provider's reticence in talking with parents about the consultant's involvement. The consultant thinks with providers about their relationship with the family and ways to overcome the mutual mistrust or antagonism that would prohibit the consultant's involvement and interfere with the adults' communication about the child. Only as all of the adults involved in the child's life truly trust the others' intentions can they engage in the process of considering the child's experience and needs.

Parent Involvement

Beyond fostering a sense of collaboration and gaining trust, the purpose of the consultant's initial meetings with parents is to elicit information they alone possess about their child. Only as conversations with parents suggest a need for fuller exploration and assistance does she offer on-going involvement. The extent of the consultant's involvement with families and the focus of their work together evolve organically. The length and breadth of the relationship is dependent on many factors including: the parent's interest and ability to participate and the intensity and severity of the child's needs.

Proposing extended interaction or specific kinds of intervention makes sense to a parent at the point at which *they* identify a need. Even then, seeing the need is not enough. Trust in the consultant's ability to help must also have developed. So the consultant begins with a narrow focus but is ready to widen her inquiry. Suggesting limitless interaction with parents who are apprehensive or uncertain about the purpose of meeting at all would be akin to proposing marriage to someone who was wary of going on a first date.

The Consultant's Initial Conversations With Parents

With the parents' agreement established, the consultant initiates contact. In these initial conversations she is hoping to set a tone of mutuality and trust while offering information about her role.

Value the parents' perspective

Whether by phone or in person, the consultant conveys that she values the parents' perspective. The consultant concentrates on getting the parents' input in three interrelated areas: their views about their child, their assessment of the current situation in child care, and their ideas about reasons for the consultant's involvement. Conveying her openness to questions and discussion, the consultant first asks how the parent understands the provider's wish for her involvement. By asking rather than assuming, the consultant addresses a parent's particular worries. Not yet knowing the parents, the consultant has no way of anticipating what she represents or how the parents' past experiences may influence their perception of the consultant. By asking parents about their views, the consultant has an opportunity to shift distortions and clarify misconceptions. She can also add factual information about the role of a consultant to child care. Her attempt at a neutral stance also affords an opportunity to observe the ways in which a parent engages others.

The introduction might go something like this: "Hello, Mr. Thompson, my name is Corina. I'm the consultant your daughter's teachers talked to you about. I know, from them, that you thought this might be a good time for me to call you at work. Are you free to talk for a few minutes?" Given permission, the consultant continues, "I'm so glad we could connect. I imagine you might be wondering who I am and how Sonia's teachers came to call on me. I know you and the teachers talked about their wish for my involvement. From that conversation did you come up with some ideas about me, or did it create some questions I could answer?"

Raising three young daughters on his own and working two jobs to support his family, Mr. Thompson has little time for small talk. He conveys even less tolerance for "agency people who butt their noses in others' business when they don't even know him or his girls." The consultant learns that his suspicion of "people who are supposed to help but mess everything up" has developed since his wife's substance abuse problem forced him to ask her to leave their home. Since then her anger at him, along with drug-induced delusions, resulted in the mother making numerous erroneous child-abuse reports. Although none of the allegations were substantiated, each led to lengthy investigations. Understandably, Mr. Thompson has come to regard outside "helpers" negatively. By beginning with inquiry rather than assumptions, the consultant learns about what underlies Mr. Thompson's hostile rebuffs of her initial overtures and is able to position herself in ways that might, over time, contradict Mr. Thompson's negative expectations. No simple explanation of the consultant's role would have sufficed.

Explore the parent's perception

Mr. Thompson held a particularly pessimistic view of helping professionals. Not all parents have such strong and solely negative ideas about who the consultant might be. Parents' past experience with helping professionals, particularly mental health professionals, effects their understanding of the consultant's role and their willingness to engage the consultant.

The consultant inquires about the parents' perception of her role and determines her direction by the parents' understanding. She may need to address parents' fears or curtail their grandiose hopes. Even when the parents' view of the consultant is unencumbered by unrealistic projections, the initial conversations allow the consultant to elaborate on how she might be involved.

Describe consultation activities

The consultant briefly describes the activities involved in case consultation. She links these interrelated efforts to the goal of assisting the child in the child-care setting and asks permission to observe their child in the child-care milieu. Her contribution is to assist the adults in putting together the pieces of the puzzle so she needs to speak with all the adults in the child's life. By sharing the knowledge each of us holds about a child, we can often develop a more comprehensive understanding and ameliorate a child's distress.

Consultation is a process. She accumulates information and assembles a picture of the child from which all of the adults in a child's life can learn and adapt their interactions on his or her behalf. The consultant contributes a specific expertise—knowledge about young children and about child care. Simultaneously, the consultant acknowledges the parents' particular and incomparable knowledge of their child.

Understanding From the Parents' Perspective

The consultant's general description of her role segues into inquiry about the parents' perceptions about their child, the specific concerns that precipitated the request for consultation, and the child-care providers' efforts. The consultant identifies her desire to gain from the parents' perspective, not to judge it or them. Somewhere in these opening encounters, the consultant suggests that she would welcome meeting with the parents to learn more about their ideas and about their child. She might do so by offering, "While I am sure that I will get some sense of Billy from his teachers and from watching how things go for him at child care, I imagine I could have a much fuller picture of your son if you could help me to get to know him."

The consultant's introductory conversations with parents often focuses on getting a sense of what they make of the teachers' questions or concerns. The consultant asks directly for the parents' ideas and explanation regarding the particular behaviors or experiences of their child in child care which precipitated the request for consultation. She is also likely to hear about the parents' view of the child-care setting and the providers. All are vital in assessing the provider–parent relationship: the differences in experience and perception of the child at home and child care, the level of distress, and the openness to the consultant's involvement.

The consultant communicates that perceptions are meaningful without conferring validity or disconfirming accuracy. Through this stance, she is proposing that deeper understanding is not gained by accumulating "facts" but by exploring how views about a child have developed. Therefore, understanding begins to be seen as a process.

Case Example

We rejoin the staff of Good Days Child Care Center as they resume thinking about Justin. Freed from the conflicts that clouded consideration, the staff's attention turns to Justin and the process of engaging his guardian, his grandmother Mrs. Jones.

> Several weeks after the initial conversation about the providers' wish to begin consultation around Justin, the idea of engaging his grandmother resurfaced. The tenor of the discussion was quite different than the previous one. With little hope that Mrs. Jones would talk to the consultant, the staff cooperatively decided that Sue would initiate the conversation with her.
>
> The three teachers shared their perceptions of Mrs. Jones and how they imagined she would receive the invitation for consultation. They believed that

Mrs. Jones was "the culprit" responsible for Justin's difficulties. They characterized her care of Justin as inconsistent: "She's all over him one minute and then could forget he's here on another day." When asked about the possibility that Mrs. Jones might be an ally in assisting Justin, Latania voiced her apprehension, "How can she help us, she can barely be there for him."

The consultant reflected the staff's discouragement, "So it sounds like you're not sure Justin can count on his grandmother, making it doubly difficult for all of you to imagine she will be a partner in figuring out how to help him at school." Empathizing first with the staff's lack of optimism, the consultant goes on to convey her desire to involve Justin's grandmother.

Sue spoke with Mrs. Jones. She described the staff's wish for the consultant's help in easing Justin's difficulties in child care. Having practiced with the consultant for these conversations, Sue confidently conveyed information about consultation. Sue also communicated the importance of Mrs. Jones' involvement in the process of understanding and helping Justin.

Mrs. Jones welcomed the consultant's involvement with the staff. However, she did not see her own participation as necessary. Besides, she added she was "way too busy to be running to more meetings about Little J." Prior experience of consultation and knowing Mrs. Jones prepared Sue for the half-hearted acceptance. Given the preparatory conversation with the consultant, Sue refrained from retaliating defensively to Mrs. Jones' inference that the staff, not she, needed help with Justin. Sue acknowledged Mrs. Jones' feeling overwhelmed by another demand on her time. Without being detoured by the need to defend her own competence, Sue persevered. She talked about the need for Mrs. Jones' involvement as it related to her position as the most important and knowledgeable person about Justin. Sue added that neither she nor the consultant wanted to add to Mrs. Jones' burden and wondered if a phone call from the consultant would be the easiest way to begin.

With Mrs. Jones' permission, the consultant called her. The wires were their exclusive mode of communication for several weeks. Initially, the consultant wondered if Mrs. Jones had questions about who she was and why the teachers had requested her involvement. Knowing that mental health consultation would be an unfamiliar service and might raise worries and suspicion, the consultant carefully considered and responded to Mrs. Jones' many queries, particularly her worries about the words "mental health."

The consultant let Mrs. Jones know about her background with a range of children and acknowledged the connotation of her title: Mental Health Consultant often, but not in this case, inferred the opposite—mental illness. She also told Mrs. Jones about her longstanding relationship with the center to quell her fears that Justin was singled out. Focusing on Justin was an attempt to ensure that his experience at Good Days was optimal. Accepting this explanation, Mrs. Jones was still not convinced that her inclusion was necessary. In response, the consultant spoke about her and the providers' limits. Without Mrs. Jones' help they would quickly encounter roadblocks to providing the quality care that the providers and Justin's grandmother wanted.

By the end of several conversations, Mrs. Jones seemed satisfied that the consultant was not called in to label her grandson "crazy." The consultant was also able to convey that Mrs. Jones' view was central to understanding Justin. Mrs. Jones gave permission to observe Justin and agreed to meet with the consultant. Undoubtedly, the first face-to-face meeting was encouraged by the consultant's offer to meet Mrs. Jones at her job.

During this phase of consultation, the consultant's energies were primarily directed at demonstrating her appreciation of all the adults' subjective experience. She wondered about their sense of her, of Justin, and of each other. First the consultant attended to the providers' assumptions about Mrs. Jones in preparing for the consultation invitation. Knowing the providers' views of Mrs. Jones also helped the consultant anticipate how she would be received. Alerted to the possibility that the grandmother might have reciprocal feelings of mistrust and blame, the consultant prepared Sue and herself for Mrs. Jones' reluctance. She was ready to disconfirm Mrs. Jones' negative expectations in word and action and hoped to repair the fractured parent–staff relationship.

Summary

As a request for case consultation emerges, the consultant considers and responds to the reasons for its arrival. A child's distress or developmental difficulties may alert providers to the need or alternately serve as a catalyst for considering dysfunction in the broader child-care community. Either alternative calls for the consultant's attention to both the child and the system in which he is functioning and to which he is responding. The consultative capacity to continually shift between and rebalance attention allows for inclusive consideration of the child.

Inclusivity is the hallmark of case consultation. To this end, the consultant engages the child's parents from the beginning, asserting the centrality of their position, and cultivating their involvement. Fostering parents' ability to offer the essential information, the consultant explores and honors their perceptions and opinions about their child.

The tone of consultation is set in this initial phase. The consultant has established who is involved, how ideas are elicited, and respect for a range of subjective experience.

Chapter 7

Gathering Information and Creating a Picture of the Child

C ase consultation was launched in the previous chapter. The child-care program's request was registered. The consultant's flexible traversing between programmatic obstacles and child-focused concerns removed impediments to initiation. The essential participants—providers and parents—were introduced to the process, and permission was given to focus on and observe a child.

With parents and providers on board, the consultant travels to the next phase of consultation. Observation is often the first stop, but the consultant must prepare providers for her presence, anticipating her vantage point as an observer. Therefore, we consider the unique aspects of observation from a mental health perspective.

Two additional avenues of learning about a child are explored. Case consultation draws heavily on the providers' and parents' information and knowledge of a child. The consultant's stance is crucial to gathering this information through wondering, not knowing and holding the adult's subjective experience of the child. Because adults will have varied perspectives about a child, the consultant assists then in sharing these views as neutrally as possible. Applying a nonpartisan stance, the consultant can free parents and providers from the impasse of opposing ideas, helping them unite around the common cause of understanding the child. At the conclusion of this chapter, we see the adults in our case example approach this goal on Justin's behalf.

The Perspective of the Observer

Like all of our work, observation is anchored in a transactional view of development. This theoretical lens orients our gaze and influences the hypotheses we develop. Because development is a dynamic relational process in which children are active contributors, the quality of relationships impacts the child's development, and the child's way of being in the world affects the caregiver's response. Observation focuses not just on the child but on what goes on *between* the child and others, paying particular attention to the child's way of relating with adults. The consultant also marks the caregivers' responses. The relational view influences hypotheses about the meaning of a child's behavior and the adults' behavior. As she watches, the consultant is asking herself, "What might this child's actions and ways of engaging tell us about his view of himself and the world?" Her question is based on the belief that through an accumulation of relational experience each person develops ideas about who he is and how the world is.

She adds to her understanding the knowledge and perspective of the parents and providers—essential informants. The meaning of observation depends on their input, and its usefulness depends on their investment and thus inclusion in the process. Consequently, the consultant continues to consider the effect of her presence on the adults and children in the setting. She prepares them for her added role by defining the purpose and limits of observation.

The consultant also considers her own biases. Her personal and theoretical perceptions influence interpretation of meaning which is why awareness of early childhood education and infant mental health are advantageous. Early childhood group care experience exposes the consultant to child-care curricula and philosophies, methods of observation and assessment, and knowledge of early childhood development. Each is necessary for understanding the demands on children and adults in the child-care setting and for moving toward a more comprehensive picture of a child's and his caregivers' challenges.

Purposes of Child Observation

The Child's Way of Relating

Observation offers the opportunity to collect particular pieces of information about a child's functioning. The consultant has limited knowledge of the child she is observing and must combine her observations with knowledge from other sources, specifically providers' and parents' longstanding and fulsome perceptions of a child. She uses these components to assess a child's abilities, limitations, vulnerabilities, and strengths. In the group milieu, the consultant sees exchanges between the child and peers and between the child and adults. This provides the consultant with some sense of the child's social style and ways of relating.

The Adult's Response

From watching interactions over time, the consultant surmises some about the providers' feelings about and perceptions of the child. She also begins to identify adult interactions and responses that are useful to the child and those that lack efficacy. While painfully aware of efforts that don't work, providers often overlook the responses that remedy a child's distress. The consultant has an opportunity to also note these actions of assistance and use them to enhance the provider–child relationships.

The Environment

The consultant opens the aperture of her observational lens wider to include the program. As she observes, she takes note of routines and program practices and asks herself these questions: Is play emphasized or do preacademic activities predominate? Are transitions anticipated? Are activities explained? She looks at how the physical environment is set up. Are there opportunities for quiet as well as active play? Is the environment structured such that children can clearly identify what is expected in each area?

Just as observation offers an avenue of insight into a child, it supplies data about a program. The consultant gets a first-hand glimpse of a program's philosophy in action and a unique peek at a provider's skills and sensitivities. Rather than rating the program, the consultant is assessing the goodness of fit between its characteristics and the child's needs and capacities. An unstructured program in which activity is self-initiated may suit most children well. The same setting may disorganize and overwhelm a child who lacks play ideas and easily becomes unregulated.

Observer Position

The luxury of being uninvolved in interactions at times allows the consultant to identify antecedents to behavior. Seeing the peer provocation that precedes an aggressive act, or conversely seeing nothing in the external environment elicit it, provides clues to the causes of behavior. The antecedents to acting out or turning inward often go unnoticed by child-care providers. They are engaged in responding to the multiple demands of the group, which necessarily precludes sustained attention to an individual child. The consultant's singular focus can be useful in revealing additional information about the child.

Having another set of eyes see the concerns she has been trying to convey can be comforting to a provider. Promoting a provider's sense of being seen is a powerful therapeutic intervention. Observation alone does not confer such meaning so the consultant must reflect this sense to the provider.

Witnessing *with* another is often integral to feeling truly understood. Being a spectator to a child's upset and the caregivers' struggle to respond to this distress contributes to the feeling that the consultant possesses a true picture of both.

The consultant's observations take place primarily in child care as this is the setting in which she will aim to effect change. However, observing a child in other settings, particularly at home, can enhance her effort. Seeing similarities or differences in how a child feels, interacts, and behaves in various settings contributes useful data.

Preparing Providers for Observation

Observation at home or in child care begins by talking with the involved adults about the reasons for and the focus of the observation. The consultant is as interested in hearing others' ideas as she is in explaining her own agenda. The purpose is mutually pursued and determined before the consultant begins her observation. Similarly, her preferred observational stance is discussed and agreed to before she arrives.

Addressing expectations

When asked or offering to observe, the consultant wonders what the adults expect, focusing particularly on perceived outcomes related to her presence. Although most providers and parents do not express their desired outcome, they usually hope that through observation the child will begin to behave better. Child-care providers allude to this fantasy in the ways they request the observation. Likely seeing observation as an intervention, a provider pleads, "Can't you just observe him a few more times? I know it would help." These requests may also signal a belief that the consultant, not she, is the agent of change. The hope that the consultant's waving a magic wand will transform the child may also represent the providers' feelings of helplessness and desperation. The consultant tries to curtail the providers' misplaced hopes and fantasies. If unattended to, these unrealistic expectations can obscure the true power of observation.

While freeing providers of their misconceptions, the consultant is careful to empathize with the underlying feelings. The consultant acknowledges the providers' panic or pain at being unable to relieve a child's misery. While communicating empathy, the consultant voices an alternate idea about the usefulness of observation. She communicates this by saying something like, "If having my eyes on Elijah could help him begin to play or speak more, I'd gladly leave this pair of peepers with you. Unfortunately, I think it's going to take more than that from all of us, especially all of you who are far more influential than I will ever be. But I surely appreciate the wish for an easy solution to his problems, especially given how concerned you are about his development. I know it's little consolation, but I can suggest some ideas about how observation can benefit us."

Defining purpose

The observational rationale is explained in relation to the specific child and in ways that will make sense to the providers. Given permission to present her intentions, the consultant might continue, "I don't want to give the impression that I think observing him will be of no use. I will observe repeatedly if we decide that is what's needed to get a handle on what's interfering with his developing in the ways we would expect of a 19-month-old. I agree that having an extra pair of eyes fixed on Elijah could provide us some clues, especially since I have the luxury of looking at him exclusively and you're having to attend to so much in addition to him. After I observe, we'll put our heads together and see if my observations offer any additional insights. I know it feels frustrating, but from what you have told me about Elijah I think you already hold many parts of the puzzle to understanding him. I hope my observations add a few more pieces. Then we'll work on assembling all our bits into a clearer picture."

The consultant explains how observation can assist in the effort of understanding a child, underscoring the mutuality of the endeavor. She places the power back where it belongs with the caregivers. If understanding is to occur or if gains are made with the child, it will have been primarily the caregivers' doing. Of course, the consultant will contribute.

Planning observation time and focus

The consultant entertains and responds to the providers' ideas about optimal times to observe and directs her attention to the aspects of the child that they have identified. The frequency and timing of observations are based on several factors: The caregivers' convenience and their view of when the consultant is most likely to witness the concerning behaviors are the most important. The consultant's presence at these times underscores her appreciation of the providers' knowledge of the child. Giving providers control over the consultant's presence also demonstrates respect. When providers choose the timing of observations and can anticipate the consultant's arrival, they are usually more comfortable in her presence. Seeing providers behave in their usual fashion ensures the reliability of the observation.

Considering the child's response

The mere presence of an outsider may influence a child's behavior. Noticing a child more intently or immediately than usual frequently elicits a new response or prevents old behaviors. If the child is expressly pointed out or alerted in advance to the fact that they are the focus of the consultant's attention, the child will most likely behave differently. Predicting this possible outcome, the consultant talks with the child's parents, as well as with the providers, about the potential adverse effect of drawing attention to the child as the specific subject of the consultant's watchful eye.

Preparing the classroom's children

Accounting for the consultant's presence in the classroom becomes a question. The consultant suggests being introduced as a visitor because in fact she is. She then asks how children are made aware of other visitors to the center. The consultant takes her cue from the providers and establishes herself on the basis of their wishes and the program's protocol, but the very conversation offers information about how the children's experience is considered. Over time, the consultant may become a familiar presence in the center so this detailed discussion need only occur around the first few visits.

Preparing the providers

The consultant prepares the providers for her plan to be an unobtrusive observer. This is not meant to suggest that the consultant sits affectless or that she never interacts. However, she is attempting to position herself so that she is free to follow and focus on the child she is observing. Because this removed stance invites misperceptions, she explains how it benefits the overall effort of learning about the child. She does not want providers to interpret her lack of involvement as disinterest or to feel that her remove represents a sense of elevated status. Providers may be inhibited or feel compelled to perform. The consultant's presence can also raise the providers' awareness of the child she is there to see and change the interaction.

She also hopes to enlist the providers' assistance in maintaining an unobstructed view of the child she is observing. She knows that any hope of steering clear of entanglement and interruptions depends on the providers. On occasion, interaction is called for, either as a way of learning more about a child or to promote or preserve her relationship with providers.

If a consultant plans to record observations, she wants to anticipate note-taking with the providers. In explaining her reasoning for documenting observations, she can avert intimidating providers or raising their suspicions. Based on interactions with previous observers, they may fear negative evaluations or scrutiny. By offering to share observational notes with the providers, the consultant can genuinely reassure them of her intentions. This offer is not solely a show of good faith. Engaging providers in reflecting on observational recording is actually a reason for writing them. The consultant explains that, by transcribing her observations, she will retain a fuller picture of what she has seen.

How and What to Observe

Thoughtfully and everything, respectively, are the obvious answers to the questions how and what is the consultant observing. Articulating the more refined aspects of positioning and focus strengthens the consultant's observational skills and exemplifies the purpose of observation for providers.

Responses to an outsider

The children, the providers, and the identified child are all affected by the consultant's presence. Children's curiosity about a new person is expected. How the children engage the consultant and how many approach her is informative. When the tone of a classroom is responsive, children are generally secure in their relationships. They are curious about an unfamiliar person but not intensely in need of her approval or interaction. Indiscriminant approaches and desperate bids for attention by many children suggest a different classroom climate. The consultant stores this information as it may be linked to the experience of the child she is observing.

Possible interactions

Invariably, the consultant engages with the children. She acknowledges children's overtures, but she does not prolong the interaction. She balances a wish to be responsive to all the children with the need to track the child she is observing. She extricates herself from lengthy interactions by answering children's questions and redirecting them. In response to inquiries about who she is and what she is doing, a consultant could respond, "I came to see what children in your school do. What (or who) do you like to play with?" This simple statement is often enough to appease children's wondering. The inquiry at the end of this statement can reconnect a child with an enjoyed activity or preferred playmate, freeing the consultant to reestablish focus.

Responding to affect

Although she does not actively participate, the consultant is responsive. In the observational context, the consultant shows interest in children and providers through small gestures and affective expressions. A smile and soft clap acknowledges a child's ascent to the top of a climbing structure. Mimicking rotating movements during a rendition of "The Wheels on the Bus" goes far toward gaining a provider's confidence that the consultant knows something about child care. Retrieving an out-of-reach bottle for a caregiver whose hands are full shows that the consultant is attentive and sensitive to the constant demands of group care.

Whether the consultant is engaging or sitting silently, she maintains an awareness of her impact on children and staff. Her actions, no matter how slight, are meaningful particularly to the providers. She is keenly attuned to how her responses influence the providers' view of her. As a guest in the providers' environment, she asks permission and inquires about and follows rules and routines.

Interacting at request

Although usually an unobtrusive observer, the consultant may become more actively engaged. When invited to act, the consultant carefully weighs the effect of accepting or declining. Assessing that her involvement puts providers at ease or conveys respect, the consultant participates. Even when involved, the consultant defers to those in charge, looking for instruction from and directing children to providers as the experts in their environment.

Interacting with the child

In limited circumstances, the consultant interacts with the child she is observing. Direct interaction is useful when what is naturally occurring between providers and the child doesn't afford the consultant the opportunity to accurately assess a child's capacities. Usually these are instances in which some aspect of the child's developmental functioning is not easily identifiable in the course of naturalistic observation. Like subtle processing problems or specific cognitive concerns may not reveal themselves. The consultant doesn't immediately insert herself.

After a few observations the consultant develops a tentative theory about the child's functioning. Needing more data to test her hypothesis, the consultant asks the providers' assistance in getting a clearer picture. When wondering about an auditory processing problem, the consultant wants to see if replacing verbal instruction with visual cuing increases a child's ability to respond appropriately. The consultant starts by sharing her theory with providers. In conversations during staff meetings, she states her idea, "I noticed Ricardo having a lot of trouble following directions. Like when you were telling him what he needed to do to be ready to go outside, the words seemed to confuse, rather than clarify, things for him. When he doesn't do what you ask him to, I'm sure it's frustrating. I know you see his misbehavior as willful, but having watched him for a while I don't think he's intentionally ignoring you. I suspect he has difficulty making sense of your words. If you're willing to, we could test out my idea. Could you use pictures or gestures along with talking to him?"

If providers are able to enact the ideas, the assessment process continues. When the providers are unable to act as instruments of assessment, the consultant considers direct involvement. She gets the staff's permission to do so. She also talks with them about how her interaction benefits the overall effort of understanding the child.

Assuming that the consultant's direct involvement is needed in the above vignette, she could acquire the staff's permission and state her desire by saying, "I don't think we've been able to test out my theory about Ricardo. You're telling me that it's been hard to find time to try the visual cues we talked about. If he learns better by show rather than tell, he's not unique. Lots of us benefit from being shown, not just told, what to do. If you think it would be helpful, I'd be happy to demonstrate what I mean by visual cues. You'd have a chance to see what I was talking about, and I'd have an opportunity to test my theory. Since this will be an artificial situation, I'm sure he will respond differently to me than he would if you were doing the same things. Second, I know that the concentrated one-on-one time that I am able to offer is not a realistic expectation of you, but I hope our experiment gives us some clues." With the child-care staff's permission and consensus that her action benefits their effort, the consultant moves from observation to interaction.

Watching and Recording

A simple narrative format works well for chronicling observation (see Figure 1). The consultant incrementally records a description of what she sees the child doing in as much detail as possible. Although this seems straightforward, the trick is capturing what one sees without interpretation. The consultant refrains from, or is at least aware of adding, inference. When watching a child, she writes: "Stephanie turns away from the caregiver who is approaching her. She clings to her mother, burying her face in the folds of her mother's skirt." The consultant does not interpret Stephanie's behavior as a sure sign of shyness. When describing the action of another child, she does not attribute aggressive intention; instead she notes, "Celeste simultaneously raises her fist and outstretches her leg toward a child who enters the dramatic play area." The causes and meaning of behavior are myriad and are not found in the behavior itself. Rather, meaning is created by synthesizing information from many sources over time.

Case Example

At the caregivers' request the consultant arrives mid-morning for the first of several observations of Justin. Passing through the center's entry way, she is immediately surrounded by a gaggle of 2- and 3-year-olds being readied for a walk to the nearby park. In the flurry, the consultant spots Justin wedged in his cubby. His little legs flail about, occasionally connecting with a passerby. Squeals and screams erupt from both Justin and his seemingly unintended targets. The commotion catches the attention of one of the caregivers.

Figure 1

Child Observation: Domains and Questions

Sense of Self

- What does the child expect of him or herself? Is the child able to make his or her needs and wants known to others? Does the child seem competent, confident, helpless? Can the child have an effect?

- Does the child take pleasure in abilities, accomplishments, interactions?

- Is the child able to self-comfort?

Affective Expression

- Does the child have a range of affect?

- What is the child's response to disappointment, frustration, pleasure?

- How flexibly does the child shift moods or affective states?

- Are affective responses and their intensity appropriate to the situation?

- What is the child's characteristic way of responding to new situations, transitions, disappointment, frustration, adult requests, and instruction?

Relationships With Adults

- What does the child's behavior say about her or his expectations of adults? (e.g., I expect: comfort, help, pleasure or disregard, disdain, punishment)

Continues on next page

Figure 1

Child Observation: Domains and Questions *(cont'd)*

- How does the child use adults? Seldom seeks out or avoids the adult; passively accepts what is offered; gives up or persists in making needs known; is involved in and takes pleasure in interactions?

- What types of interaction does the child respond to? What does the adult do to organize, comfort, guide, clarify?

Communication or Language

- How is expression or language used? (e.g., to make needs or wants known, to plan, to problem solve, to get information, to express ideas, and/or to recall experience)

- Is expressiveness/speech expectable for the child's age and experience?

- What cognitive characteristics are reflected in how language is used? (e.g., spontaneous, repetitive, limited repertoire, rigid, flexible, and/or self-stimulating or soothing)

Motor Capacities

- How does the child use her or his body given the child's age and experiences?

- What are the characteristics of movement? Is the child agile, tentative, clumsy, awkward, coordinated?

- Is the child aware of her or his body in space? (e.g., navigates easily or bumps into objects or others)

Continues on next page

Figure 1

Child Observation: Domains and Questions *(cont'd)*

Sensory/Regulatory Capacities

- What is the child's energy level?

- What is needed to engage and maintain the child's interest? (e.g., a great deal of stimulus and/or specific types of sensory stimulus)

- What is the effect of sensory input? How does the child respond to gentle touch, deep pressure, or swaddling? What is the child's response to loud noises, lots of activity, and various types of tactile stimulation?

Relationship to and Participation in the Group

- How does the child respond to group activities?

- How does the child respond to group instruction/direction?

- How does the child respond to transitions or changes in routine?

- Is the child interested in particular objects, activities, peers?

- In what types of play/activities is the child involved? Is the child interested in a range of activities or consistently involved in only one type? Does the child take pleasure in play? Are play themes easily extendable or rigid and perseverative? What contributes to the child's choices of where and with whom to engage?

Bending down to meet Justin's gaze, the provider, Latania, tries to cajole him from his secure spot. Gently she implores, "Come on little man, you know we go to the park every day after snack." Not persuaded by this reminder, Justin covers his eyes and burrows in. Turning an upward grimace to the consultant, Latania whispers, "This is a daily deal, it's getting old." With a nod, the consultant conveys sympathy for Latania's struggle.

Eventually able to extract Justin from his hiding place, Latania helps him with his coat and carries him to meet the haphazardly assembled group at the sidewalk. Justin looks comfortable settled in the crux of his caregiver's arms. Suddenly spying the consultant, Justin scowls and sputters, "No, go away, bad lady." His attempts to banish her intensify as he bats his hands in the consultant's direction. Wanting to acknowledge the fear that seems to underlie Justin's response, the consultant backs away. Noticing Latania looking quizzical and confused by both Justin's and her own actions, the consultant adds, "I'm a new person to this little fellow. Latania, how shall we let him and the others know who I am and, probably more to the point, who I'm not?" The carefully prepared introduction of the consultant was forgotten in the chaos of the moment. The consultant's comment is a gentle reminder, tailored to Justin's response to her presence. The prompt is lost on Latania so the consultant takes the lead. On their walk, the consultant speaks simply to all who are interested. Justin watches wide eyed and listens intently. "I came to see your school. I'm going to watch you all play at the park. I will be at your school while you eat lunch and then I'll say good-bye when you lay down to rest. I'm not a new teacher. Your teachers will stay with you, and I will go home." Directing her closing comment to Justin, the consultant concludes. "When we get to the park, I'll sit on the bench. I won't get too close because you don't know me yet."

When they reach the park, the consultant positions herself as promised. She jots notes hastily, hoping to capture what she has seen so far but not wanting to miss what is currently occurring. She records Justin's struggle with the transition as well as his response to an unfamiliar face. Sensing a set of eyes on her, the consultant looks up from her writing. Justin sits frozen in the sandbox where Latania deposited him. His gaze is fixed upon her. Hoping to convey comfort, she smiles. Justin averts his eyes but remains motionless.

Sue, the senior provider, joins Justin in the sandbox. Placing a pail between his outstretched legs, she tries to entice him into interaction, scooping shovels of sand and depositing them in the bucket's bottom. She quizzes, "Justin want more? Want to fill it up yourself?" Justin is not distracted. Sue shrugs her uncertainty to the consultant.

A few minutes later, Sue sits down next to the consultant and verbalizes her confusion, "That's odd, I haven't seen him that still in ages." The consultant asks, "I guess I'm not seeing a typical time at the park for Justin? How about the transition, was that similar to what you usually experience?" She receives the confirmation she expects. The tumultuous transition was typical, while the stillness is unusual.

Knowing that an upcoming meeting will afford time for a more fulsome discussion with all the staff, the consultant plants a seed for consideration: "It's really helpful for me to hear about the similarities and differences between what I see and what you all experience everyday. We'll ponder the reasons as we go along, but I'm especially curious about the stone-statue response, especially since you're telling me it's not Justin's usual way. It seemed like when he saw me, a stranger, he got scared, literally scared stiff. I'm struck by the similarity to your description of his behavior when he started at the center, when everyone was unfamiliar. I wonder if we're hitting on something important about what newness feels like to Justin." Intrigued by the possible connection, Sue was eager to talk with her coworkers. Sue suddenly bolts from the bench toward the spray of sand and tangled clump of toddlers in the sandbox.

Sitting atop one sand-covered child, Justin wrestled with another for possession of a shovel. Sue dislodged the sand toy and freed the pinned prisoner while recounting Justin's indiscretions, "You can't hurt kids. You have to share. Besides," she reminded him, "you didn't want that shovel. You weren't even using it."

On the face of it, Sue's admonishments were accurate, but the consultant wondered if possession, not play, was Justin's priority. Vigilance seemed to take precedence for Justin. Maybe he couldn't afford to explore the properties of conservation when preoccupied by the potentially threatening activities of an unpredictable stranger.

Sue separated a crying Justin from his peers, telling him his reentry to the group was contingent on his ability to share. Just as Justin stopped sobbing and had begun to play, it was time to return to the center. Without much warning, toys were scooped up, and children were shepherded toward the street. The sudden shift shook Justin's tenuously attained equilibrium. Seeing Tometrius approaching, Justin sprang upright and trotted toward the climbing structure.

Justin sequestered himself in a nook too tiny for adults to enter. Tometrius patiently pleaded and then firmly demanded he abandon his bunker. Finally exasperated, she turns and walks away. Seeing her retreat, Justin pops from his hiding place and, with what seems to the consultant like panic, he repeatedly implores, "No go." Throwing his tiny torso to the ground, Justin cries quietly for "mommy," bringing Tometrius back.

Clearly conflicted, the caregiver steadies Justin to his feet and coaxes him to walk. As the distressed duo passes, Tometrius offers an aside: "We agreed he has to walk like the other kids, but I'm the only one who sticks with the plan. Look at the reward—I get to be the bad guy." Registering Tometrius' complaint, the consultant makes a mental note. With Tometrius' permission, she will bring up the disagreement for discussion during the next staff meeting.

Everyone's exhaustion, mixed with dissension among the staff, makes for a miserable return walk to the center. Reaching the room, a chorus of crying children rush to tables not yet outfitted with the noon meal. Sue snaps at the other two providers to speed up as she places meatloaf, mounds of mashed potatoes, and bowls of lukewarm legumes on each of three tables. Latania takes charge of toileting. Tometrius, still fuming, takes her time. From the bathroom, Latania loudly reports: "He wet himself again," referring to Justin. She adds, this time talking about Justin's grandmother, "and you know she didn't bring that change of clothes we asked for."

Appearing in pants that are clearly too big, Justin pulls at the droopy dungarees and whines, "No Granny's," seeming to signal yet again that the unfamiliar is unwanted. The necessary change in attire makes Justin last to lunch, aggravating his already unstable mood. Sue, his primary caregiver, shows Justin there is plenty for everyone to eat, yet Justin tries to take food from others' plates. He grabs for a glass of milk mid-pour, sending a lake of liquid into the bowl of beans. Finally, seeing his plate is still empty, he flings it Frisbee-style, grazing Sue's cheek. Sue stands, "That's it, Justin; we'll try again later. You need to calm down." With a loose grip on Justin and on her anger, Sue whisks Justin out of his seat. Sue's path crosses the consultants'. Suddenly, mad morphs into embarrassment. Compelled to explain her uncharacteristically harsh response, Sue sputters, "Sorry, but I've got to get him out of here before he really hurts somebody." The consultant tries to console Sue, "No, I'm sorry for you and Justin; this is really hard on both of you."

By the time Sue is out of sight, anarchy has erupted at her unattended table. Without Sue's solid presence, the children and her less experienced colleagues are untethered. Quickly considering the cost–benefit balance, the consultant asks if she can assist. The offer is met with palpable relief. Settling herself on a pint-sized seat, the consultant reintroduces herself to the group. Asking for instruction about the lunchtime routine, she falls into the flow of activity.

Ladling last helpings and wiping faces, the consultant sees Sue's surprise as she returns unaccompanied by Justin. Trying to read the response, she explains, "I couldn't fill your shoes, but filling plates is a bit of help, I hope?" Assured of being irreplaceable, Sue seems genuinely appreciative.

Wondering about Justin, the consultant learns he is in an adjoining quiet area. Sue hopes that he has fallen asleep from exhaustion. Questions reveal that isolating Justin from the group is common. Ill at ease with both what she hears and how to address it in the moment, the consultant sits quietly and formulates her response.

Interrupted by the assembling of cots that signals naptime is near, the consultant recognizes it is time for her to leave. Preparing everyone for her departure, she makes the rounds saying good-bye to children and providers. Sitting down beside Sue, she wonders, "Do you think checking on Justin before I go is an okay idea? He seems so attuned to comings and goings and so sensitive to strangers, I don't want to disappear. I don't think it's me that matters but maybe what I represent. Could we look in on him together? I'm sure knowing you're around is what's important." Reminded of her centrality and seeing the logic in this suggestion, Sue and the consultant adjourn to the adjacent area where a groggy Justin is gathered up by Sue and rocked gently as the consultant bids them both good-bye.

The value of observing is evident in this single snapshot. Watching Justin's apprehension at the unfamiliar and his struggles with transitions, the consultant is asking, "What do these responses tell me about his expectations of the world, and relationships?" She entertains multiple meanings and formulates questions to confirm or disallow percolating theories.

The inquiries she generates will, for the most part, wait to be tested. However, she experiments with a few in the moment. She wonders with Sue if Justin's paralysis represents an extreme fear of the unknown. By questioning the practice of leaving Justin alone, the consultant introduces separations and loss and comings and goings as possible contributors to Justin's concerning behavior.

The consultant's adherence to transaction extends beyond Justin. She collects information coming from the providers and the child regarding their evolving experiences of themselves, of each other, and of her. The consultant conveys her underlying intention because she knows that her actions will be interpreted. In observation, affective expression is relied on heavily. The consultant signaled sympathy with a nod and offered support with a smile. Occasionally, she was able to express intention verbally. She is careful not to burden providers when they are busy or to usurp the importance of attending to children by engaging in long conversations. With or without words, the consultant took every opportunity to confirm the providers' reality. However, she does not do so at Justin's expense, speaking equally to his and the providers' subjective experiences. The consultant remained removed until she saw a spot where inaction would likely be interpreted as disregard. Even as she offered assistance at the lunch table, she prepared to right the balance based on Sue's response.

The consultant seeks clarity without conferring judgment. A consultant who approached observation as a way of determining what was "wrong" with Justin or in what ways the providers' efforts were "failing" would be doing a disservice to all if she were to draw conclusions from a single observation. That things are not going well for Justin and his providers is clear, but why each is struggling is as yet unknown. As the observation is added to information obtained in future visits, as well as conversation with all the adults, we will come to a clearer understanding of the contributors and how to address them.

Reflecting on the Observation

Information gleaned from observations becomes useful only as providers incorporate it into their developing understanding of the child. Providers accept this information if they feel the consultant possesses a representative picture and appreciates what they typically experience. Therefore, the consultant verifies her observations. At the end of one observation or after several, the consultant asks, "Was this the way days usually go?" or "Do you think I've been here enough to get a clear picture of him?" The consultant acknowledges that her view is limited. As observation is necessarily intermittent and anecdotal, the consultant doesn't expect to possess the providers' panoramic perspective.

Examining Variations

Observations yield useful information even when the consultant does not see how a child usually functions. The consultant is interested in what accounts for the difference. Providers often attribute the shifts solely to the consultant's presence. By inference, her consistent presence is the only solution to the problem. Knowing she does not possess magical power, the consultant is not satisfied with the explanation; however, she entertains the possibility that her watchful eye has an impact. The consultant asks providers to consider other possibilities for shifts in behavior. Did they interact more or differently with the child when the consultant observed? Were routines or activities amended? Were staffing or group size different? These factors may offer clues to understanding and assisting the child. (If the circumstances of her observation can be replicated, the child's needs may be met.)

Confirming Subjective Experience

Observation is more immediately useful when the providers recognize the consultant's image of the child. Having established that they are looking at the same picture, they compare interpretations. From a shared vantage point, the consultant can better appreciate the providers' subjective experience of a child. She can begin to make sense of the meaning they ascribe to the child's behavior and link it to what she witnesses. For instance, she might ask, "When you picked up Phillip to take him to the changing table, I noticed he arched his back and made movements with his hands—is that the behavior that makes you wonder if he has some type of autistic disorder? You were telling me you've been concerned ever since you read about autism in your child development class."

The consultant may question the providers' perception; however, she does not discount or criticize it. She wonders how a provider arrived at the view she holds. The consultant doesn't weigh her interpretations against the providers or parents. Reflecting upon and combining these sources of information affords the greatest likelihood of developing a nuanced and accurate picture of a child from which understanding evolves.

Gathering Information From Providers

In this phase of case consultation, the consultant is gathering information about the child, responding to the caregivers' subjective experience of the child, and establishing a template for considering the meaning of the child's behavior. Gathering information from providers begins by helping them to articulate their questions and concerns. Often, an initial description of a child is suffused with subjective feelings and void of interpretation of the meaning of behavior. Asking specific questions begins the process of deepening understanding. The consultant does not expect that providers possess all the information: "I know you're really worried about Ashley. Could I ask you some questions that I hope will help us begin to clarify what's contributing to your concern? I don't expect we'll have all or even most of the answers today, but if we lay out some specific areas to consider, we can figure out how to get the information we'll need to make sense of what's going on." The consultant conveys that understanding is a process, one on which she and the providers are embarking together. (See Figure 2 for possible areas of inquiry.)

The consultant wants to elicit the provider's current notion about the child's behavior and the reasons for that view because the provider's response to behavior is determined by the meaning ascribed to it. We can only hope to amend, disabuse, or expand upon another's ideas once we fully understand the ideas and their contributors.

Figure 2

Areas of Inquiry With Providers

- When did you first notice the behaviors?

- Have you wondered about the child's behavior or development since she or he entered the program, or has something changed recently?

- Does the behavior happen all the time or is it more likely to occur at certain times? – (during particular routines, with some people and not others, when the child is faced with specific tasks/expectations)

- Can you say a bit more about what the child does that leads you to feel the child is…(e.g., "aggressive," "wild," "spoiled," "in his own world," "not able to make friends," "odd")?

- Do you have an idea about the child's life at home?

- Do you have information about previous child-care experiences? Is this the child's first time in group care?

- How does relating with the child make you feel? – (Does this child elicit: engagement, rejection, comfort, pity, anger, and/or pleasure?)

- Do you have some sense about the child's family's cultural background and values?

- Does the child's development (in one or several domains) seem similar to other children of the same age?

The consultant's conveyed appreciation of the caregiver's subjective experience of a child often diminishes defensiveness that obstructs the caregiver's ability to accurately see and respond to the child's needs. In response to the interpretation of a child's inability to share as an indication of being spoiled, the consultant empathizes with the caregiver's perception: "I imagine her grabbing toys from other children is infuriating. You constantly have to negotiate compromises where nobody is satisfied. It must feel like Amber often gets more than the other children, making her seem spoiled. Is there something in her home life that supports that idea?"

Children who are experiencing difficulties and, consequently, are difficult to care for arouse strong feelings in their caregivers. As the caregivers begin to feel that the consultant understands these feelings and is not judgmental, empathy for the child's experience often increases. Freeing providers to consider the meaning of a child's behavior is a crucial first step.

The consultant hopes her stance of wondering instills an interest in inquiry as the process through which understanding occurs. "Wondering with, not acting upon" (Jeree Pawl, 1997; personal communication) the caregivers involves them and preserves them as the holders of essential information.

Gathering Information From Parents

In her meetings with the parents, the consultant is communicating that the child's behavior in child care can be meaningfully considered only as we are able to establish its relevance in connection to all other aspects of the child's experience. To this end, the consultant asks about the child's developmental history, relational history, constitutional particularities, and the child's current functioning outside of the child-care setting. (See Figure 3 for suggestions regarding areas of inquiry with parents.) Clearly, these areas of exploration are broad. They are offered as a general framework for the consultant's consideration as exploration unfolds organically. The consultant is not "taking a development history" or asking a litany of formal questions.

Throughout the inquiry, the consultant is explicitly informing the parents of her intentions. Her questions come with explanations of *why* and *how* the information she requests expands the understanding of their child. Making intention overt diminishes suspicion and misinterpretation; consequently, the parents' willingness to share their knowledge increases.

Phoebe, a 3-year-old who has been in her child-care center for over a year, begins to vehemently protest every transition. Her displeasure at separating from her mother has suddenly skyrocketed. Armed only with this awareness and an invitation to talk, the consultant meets with Phoebe's mother. Mrs. Schuller shares the caregivers' concerns about her daughter's newly developed distress. She and the child-care providers are equally unable to account for the shift in Phoebe's behavior.

After an introductory conversation and having established that Mrs. Schuller and the providers' perspective, albeit hazy, is mutually held, the consultant asks if Phoebe or her family members have experienced any recent changes. The consultant couches the question in a brief explanation of why she is asking, "I hope my question doesn't seem too forward. I ask because the change in Phoebe's behavior was, if I understand you and the caregivers correctly, sudden and intense. Sometimes children show us their feelings about a change in one part of their life by becoming disturbed by small shifts in other areas. Their behavior can be a way of saying, 'What else will change?'"

Mrs. Schuller seriously "racked her brain" for changes because the consultant's explanation made sense. The family hadn't experienced any major disruptions, and they had ruled out any changes in the child-care center, leaving them stuck. The impasse was momentary.

The consultant pursued another area of inquiry—the intensity of Phoebe's response: "Mrs. Schuller, I know we're flummoxed by the cause of Phoebe's upset, but does her intensity surprise you?" The consultant was headed in a useful direction. Mrs. Schuller responded: "There's never been any con-

Figure 3

Areas of Inquiry With Parents

- How and when were developmental milestones achieved?

- Was the timing and the path toward mastery what the parents expected?

- What informs the parents' developmental expectations (e.g., cultural norms, past child-rearing experience, personal beliefs and values, specific literature or education)?

- Continuities and discontinuities in caregiving relationships (e.g., previous child-care experiences, foster care, loss of caregiver, shared care by extended family, single parenting, shared custody).

- Family circumstances which may impact the child (e.g., immigration, economic status, homelessness, domestic violence).

- Child's temperament (e.g., as a newborn/infant how did she or he respond to changes in routine or caregivers?) Was the infant easy to comfort? Were state changes fluid? Was she or he easy to please, adaptable, or cranky?

- Do the parents note specific constitutional particularities (e.g., sensory sensitivities, regulatory or sensory integration difficulties, idiosyncrasies in processing)?

- Specific conditions or circumstances the child has experienced? Injuries or trauma, medical conditions, hospitalizations, illness, allergies?

fusion about what pleases or displeases Phoebe. She's let me know what she wanted and what she would have no part of from the day she was born. Any change in routine and I'd hear about it for hours." The consultant verifies her understanding: "So you're saying she has always been and still is powerfully affected by any shifts? Hearing you say that Phoebe is sensitive to slight changes, I wonder if we need to recalibrate our ideas about the magnitude of change. It sounds like an almost imperceptible deviation could feel like a seismic shift to her. Does that match your sense of her?" The theory seemed possible to Mrs. Schuller.

Now the consultant and Mrs. Schuller were looking for minute variations in routine, not a major metamorphosis. Mrs. Schuller had recently changed jobs. Her new work schedule necessitated a change in Phoebe's routine. She was now picked up a half hour later from child care. The adults agreed that the tiny temporal amendment in conjunction with this child's temperament accounted for Phoebe's fitfulness.

Couching questions in explanations of how and/or why the consultant imagines information will be useful serves several purposes. The consultant includes the parent in her thinking process, honoring their role and knowledge and building trust. Her transparency enhances the parent's willingness to join in the journey of co-creating meaning. She is not randomly plucking bits of information and independently gluing conclusions together. She demonstrates her desire to incorporate everyone's view of the child and models her approach of wondering one's way toward carefully considered conclusions. Making explicit the intent of the questions prompts a parent to consider possible contributors to the child's behavior that would go unexplored.

Maintaining the Nonpartisan Stance

When providers' and parents' ideas about a child are divergent or their feelings about one another are less than ideal, a consultant can easily be caught in the conflict. Maintaining neutrality in an embattled parent–provider relationship is quite complicated, especially when the consultant seeks to know each intimately. The consultant sets her stance early.

To parents, she explains that she is enlisted by, but not a member of the staff of, the child-care center. All of her efforts are on the child's behalf. Anchored by this stance, she is able to listen and empathize with a parent's concerns, even as they differ from or are in direct opposition to those of the child-care providers. The consultant identifies how a rupture in the parent–provider relationship may be obscuring everyone's ability to understand and support the child as much as they hope.

Holding Various Views of a Child

Holding multiple and sometimes opposite views is a hallmark of the consultant's stance. Whether these differing perspectives exist among members of a child-care staff or between parents and providers, the consultant is genuinely interested in discovering the significance of these differences. Differences exist in both the existence and interpretation of behaviors. Children's behavior can vary between situations and people, offering clues to the child's challenges. Alternatively, differences in the meaning ascribed by adults to the same behavior reveal important cues to the adults' perceptions and contributors to the behavior. The consultant must first figure out which of these scenarios account for the adults' contrasting ideas.

> Embarking on such a journey with Mrs. Jaisell, the consultant asks first about the mother's sense of her 28-month-old, who is described by his providers as "in his own world"—unable to verbalize his needs, averse to affection, and wary of interaction. Intuitively aware of her son's idiosyncratic ways of relating, Mrs. Jaisell has adapted so exquisitely to his nonverbal cues that she is in a quandary about the child-care providers' alarm. The consultant begins by voicing the contrasting levels of concern: "Sounds, from your description of Saheed, that you and his caregivers see many of the same behaviors. So it must be pretty puzzling that they are perplexed about the

very parts of Saheed that are easy for you to understand. As you were telling me about your exhaustive search for just the right child-care setting, I was imagining that your admiration might complicate the situation; to have such a different view from people you respect is, I imagine, disconcerting. You all care deeply about Saheed and describe similar behavior, and yet your feelings are at odds with one another."

The consultant does not shy away from exploring differences but accentuates similarities between the adults' experiences of the child. By identifying agreement the consultant seeks to shore up the provider–parent relationship. She wants to preserve or establish common ground in order to strengthen the relational base upon which mutual trust and understanding can flourish. The consultant interprets each group to the other in an effort to open channels of communication between all of the adults in the child's life. In a future conversation, the consultant supports this essential alliance by speaking to the providers' intentions: "Mrs. Jaisell, now that we've met a few times and I've had the pleasure of not only hearing about but seeing you and Saheed together, I've gained a greater appreciation of how attuned you are to him. It seems so effortless for you to know exactly what Saheed wants when he makes a certain sound or gestures with his finger. You've done it for so long now that I bet it's hard to fathom that it takes a bit of work for the providers to figure out what Saheed is telling them. I know his providers are really trying. I think their worry is that even with all their dedication and sensitivity, they're not always able to understand Saheed. I know their concern feels like unnecessary alarm, but I think you all share the desire for Saheed to be cared for in the best possible way."

In this situation, as in all case consultations, the consultant begins by conveying her appreciation of the parent's perspective. After naming the parent's view, she addressed the obstacle of discrepancies between the parent's and the provider's experiences.

The consultant empathizes equally with the parent's and the providers' experiences. Understanding another's subjective experience is not synonymous with acceptance. Eventually, the consultant begins to represent each group's perceptions to the other in an attempt to untangle knots of misperception and establish commonality of purpose. The misperceptions causing obstruction can emanate from any of the adults involved—parents, providers, or the consultant herself. Wherever they originate and whenever they present themselves, they must be addressed so that the adults are free to consider the child's experience.

Case Example

We rejoin the case of Justin, as the consultant and his guardian, Mrs. Jones, are meeting face to face for the first time. In addition to gathering information to enhance everyone's understanding of Justin, the consultant finds out that she will need to address the disagreement between his grandmother and the child-care providers. A nonpartisan stance is imperative.

> Upon meeting Mrs. Jones, the consultant learned that she saw the school as the source of many of Justin's difficulties. Although Justin "wasn't always an angel at home," his grandmother saw child care as a detrimental influence. "I don't know what they're doing there, but he starts fussing as soon as we get off the bus, and by the time I leave him he's blubbering and cursing. He sure doesn't do that at my house, not anymore. It's like they got a different child at school. They say he's hitting and falling out all the time and peeing on himself."

> Quickly the consultant learns that the important adults in Justin's life, his grandmother and his child-care providers, blame the other for his increasing distress in child care. If all the adults are to work cooperatively, she will need to address the reciprocal accusations. She must first prove that she is not allied exclusively with the child-care center.

The consultant makes the first of what she knows will be many remarks aimed at establishing herself as a nonpartisan participant, "Mrs. Jones, you said that the picture the providers paint of Justin is unrecognizable. I'm hoping you can help me and his teachers solve the mystery of why he behaves differently at school. There is so much you know about Justin. Right now the teachers are grasping at straws trying to make sense of what they're seeing." Mrs. Jones is quick to capitalize on the consultant's suggestion that the providers are struggling: "They are grasping all right, but they are coming up with nothing. You'd think they'd ask me rather than trying to pull answers out of thin air." The consultant acknowledges Mrs. Jones' feelings of being dismissed. She suggests that, although the opportunity to hear from Mrs. Jones is overdue, learning about Justin now is as useful as ever.

Conveying interest in Mrs. Jones' ideas, the consultant asks, "When you were describing how Justin acts when you drop him off at child care, you added that he doesn't do that at home, 'anymore.' Was there a time when he cried and got upset like that at home?" The consultant's careful listening allows entry to Justin's past as well as current functioning.

Over the next few meetings with Mrs. Jones, the consultant learns that Justin's being caught amid tensions between his grandmother and child-care providers replicates earlier experiences. Falling through the cracks of eroded adult relationships characterized Justin's entire life. The consultant learns that Justin came into the care of Mrs. Jones, his paternal grandmother, relatively recently. She now has guardianship of him, along with three other grandchildren.

Justin is the only child from her son's union with Justin's teenage mother from whom he was removed. Although the reasons for the imposed separation are sketchy, Justin's removal is attributed to his mother's exclusion from a residential drug treatment program and suspicion of physical abuse and his father's incarceration. With neither parent available to care for him, Justin was placed with his grandmother. Since that time, Justin's mother has missed most of the scheduled visits with her son. However, she periodically arrives unannounced at the grandmother's home, often in the middle of the night. Mrs. Jones alternately attributes the sporadic nocturnal calls to her being "out of her head" or as attempts to locate Justin's father. Neither motive indicates an interest or ability to connect with Justin. Justin's mother has hampered Mrs. Jones' efforts to establish predictability regarding his mother's presence. Limited contact with his father is further constrained by the circumstances of the jail's visiting room.

Despite Mrs. Jones' valiant attempts, it is difficult for her to provide predictability and continuity for Justin. Not only is she caring for three other children, she also needs to work outside the home some weekends, leaving Justin with several, often unfamiliar, people.

Despite repeated disruption in relationships, Justin could mostly depend on his relationship with his grandmother. The consultant's appreciation of this relationship evolved during home visits at which Justin was present and through hearing his grandmother's descriptions of their interactions. As Mrs. Jones had initially asserted, Justin looked like a different child at home. He clearly communicated his needs and desires and was most often understood. He interacted playfully and at times even shared with his cousins. He asked and was helped to use the toilet, rarely having the accidents that were prevalent at child care. Although Mrs. Jones wondered how he might fare without her next to him, Justin seemed to fall asleep easily at home. The practice of falling asleep together was, she admitted, a result of her own exhaustion and not out of a sense of his need for comfort.

Witnessing Justin's disparate behaviors at home and child care broadens the consultant's sense of him. The clear differences explained, at least partially, why Mrs. Jones and the staff's relationship was filled with blame and mistrust as each held the other responsible for the behavior at child care. The staff believed that the grandmother was "in denial" or maliciously lying to them, depending on their mood and their level of frustration. Mrs. Jones felt accused and discounted by the staff. Both felt unappreciated at the time they most needed to depend on each other. Justin is, again, trapped between feuding adults.

Reconstructing the adults' relationships depends on the consultant's establishing a nonpartisan stance and simultaneously gaining Mrs. Jones' trust by demonstrating her wish to understand her subjective experience. The consultant does this by being deeply curious about Mrs. Jones' ideas. The consultant does not defend the teachers nor does she join in Mrs. Jones' accusations about them. She focuses instead on everyone's mutual interest in understanding the mystery of Justin's contrasting behavior.

By enlisting Mrs. Jones in identifying pieces of the puzzle, the consultant asserts Mrs. Jones' singular importance. The consultant elicits a comprehensive account of Justin's history. She connects it to the evolving understanding of Justin by highlighting a seemingly minor moment in their conversation. The line of inquiry that led to the unfolding of Justin's story was not fully articulated in the example. However, in this case, like all others, the consultant's questions about a child's history, development, and behavior at home were accompanied by explanations about the purpose of the questions. The consultant links the information to the goal of understanding and helping Justin.

The consultant begins to hypothesize about how the meaning of change, transition, and unpredictability in Justin's life shapes his behavior. In the next phase of consultation, she contemplates ways to usefully distill and offer the information. Certain conditions must exist for the information to be shared with and usefully incorporated by the providers. Mrs. Jones' permission is the primary condition. Therefore, the consultant explores what in their conversation can be shared and what must remain private, clarifying how and why certain information could be beneficial. The grandmother retains control of what is conveyed.

Permission from a parent, however, does not ensure the providers' acceptance of the information. The consultant must ready the ground so that the seeds of information will take root. Her task is to use her observations and the information about Justin's experience to help all the adults understand and respond to the distress that his behavior demonstrates.

Summary

Case consultation is devoted to developing a picture of the child by collecting and combining information. Providers, parents, and direct observation are viewed as equally important sources of information. Eliciting data is a skill, but integrating it is a more complex endeavor, just as assembling an intricate puzzle takes prowess beyond purchasing the pieces. Mastery at configuring a coherent picture is not enough. The consultant must make sure that everyone involved recognizes the same child, feels heard, and has given permission for the process.

Establishing an agreed-upon image of a child and engendering cooperation among all participants requires knowledge beyond development and pathology. The consultant is called on to find out about each participant's perception and how it has arisen. When discrepancies are identified or imbalances in the adults' relationships exist, the consultant is challenged to hold and represent opposing ideas while asserting collaboration as fundamental to defining and addressing the child's needs.

Chapter 8

Co-Creating Meaning—
Interpreting Behavior and
Developing Hypotheses

H aving assembled the ingredients, we turn to how meaning is made of a child's behavior in child care. A framework for interpreting and creating hypotheses about behavior is offered. The alchemy of this phase of consultation occurs as information is exchanged and synthesized. The consultant creates and holds a space in which a child's behavior can be received as meaningful communication. Creating avenues for exchange between parents and providers with the eventual aim of direct dialogue comes first. Therefore, we look at how the consultant maintains confidentiality while pursuing disclosure. Parents and providers are actively engaged in mutual articulation of the purpose of this phase of consultation. Both groups are enlisted in developing theories about the child's behavior so that they become active participants in co-creating meaning.

Sharing Information as the First Step in Co-Creating Meaning

Whether meeting conjointly or separately, the consultant engages all of the adults in the effort of co-creating meaning. By suggesting to each group that the other possesses necessary nuggets of valuable information about the child, the consultant seeks to strengthen the parent–provider relationship and encourage exchange.

When meeting with parents independent of the providers, the consultant represents their presence in the process. As she and the parents ponder possible contributors to the child's behavior, the consultant interjects information she has learned from the providers that confirms or expands the developing hypothesis.

The exchange of ideas in the effort of co-creating meaning must be reciprocal. Just as she represents the providers' ideas to the parents, the consultant ensures reciprocity by presenting what she learns from the parents to the providers. The consultant carefully assesses the impact when acting as a conduit of information regardless of directional flow. She always gains permission from parents or providers to share information or ideas. Even as she asks allowance, the consultant is aware of her ultimate goal. She seeks to promote direct communication between all of the participants in the consultative effort. The success of case consultation and, ultimately, the child rely on the supportive web of relationships in which he resides. The consultant's communications act as threads of connection between parents and providers.

A consultant may elicit information from a parent that is not yet known to the child-care provider. The consultant's positioning and stance affords opportunities to hear about the child's life in ways the providers may not be privy to. The consultant has the luxury of spending uninterrupted time with parents. Additionally, the consultant's positioning may make it easier for parents to share some types of information with her.

Her status as a mental health professional can initially be off-putting to parents. However, once the consultant gains admittance, her position can be comforting. She is an objective external participant. Standing as she does, outside the child-care structure, she has no conferred authority in relation to the parent or child. The consultant's lack of power can free parents who are fearful of sharing information that may jeopardize the child's placement or standing in the center. Also, the consultant's stance is envisaged to confer confidence and establish trust. Collectively, these characteristics cultivate parent disclosure.

When the consultant hears information that she imagines is integral to understanding the child's presentation in child care, she notes its relevance, first to herself and then to the parent. She might mark a parent's illustrative comment with an observation that something meaningful has just been shared, saying, "What you just mentioned…that Tommy regularly needs to take steroids to control his asthma, or Zhi-ling spent her first two years in Hong Kong with her grandparents, or Jesus was hospitalized several times in his infancy…seems important to our understanding of his or her experience of the world."

The consultant draws connections between the child's experience (or developmental/constitutional particularity) and his behavior in child care. The consultant makes the connection explicit. The consultant links the tentative hypothesis to the goal of improving the child's experience in child care. Fastening the evolving meaning to the child's behavior in child care reminds the parent of the consultant's primary task. She was enlisted to engage all of the adults in better understanding and thereby ameliorating the difficulties in the child-care setting.

While acknowledging the usefulness of hearing about the child from the parents' perspective, the consultant is always asserting the prominence of the parent–provider relationship as the place in which mutual understanding will best benefit the child. To this end, the consultant again expresses her view that the child-care providers would benefit greatly by walking with the parents through each step of the process.

Once parents recognize that they hold the key to access assistance for their child, they are often willing to share information with the caregivers. Parents who are excited by or proud of the discoveries they have made with the consultant's help take pleasure in "enlightening" the caregivers. At other times parents share information once they realize its relevance to their child's difficulties in child care. In these situations, information is not initially offered to providers solely because the parents are, at the time, unaware of its value.

Even when parents wish to share newfound understanding or long-held knowledge, circumstances can prevent the possibility. Logistical constraints keep parents and providers from meeting. Interpersonal issues can also interfere. Parents may feel that they lack sufficient connection with the providers to share personal information. They may worry about being judged or criticized. Parents who feel responsible for creating or contributing to their child's difficulties imagine that providers will share their view. All of these factors, or any combination, can inhibit a parent's ability to be forthcoming with providers.

The consultant appreciates and respects the parents' prohibitions, all the while persevering in opening pathways of communication. She knows that understanding is pivotal to generating the empathy that providers must possess to truly support a child. She stresses this connection; however, she offers to be the conduit of communication while expressing her desire for this role to someday be unnecessary.

Before she shares information with the providers, the consultant confirms the parents' desire for her to do so. Permission is necessary but not sufficient. The consultant rehearses with the parents what she will say to the providers. She gets confirmation that she has clearly understood the parent. For a parent who remains apprehensive about divulging sensitive information, the consultant works to find ways to say essential bits without revealing more than the parent is ready to. She assures the parent that she will extract only the parts that pertain to the child's experience. The consultant assists in distilling the information. An illustration of this delicate endeavor follows.

> A young mother is ashamed at losing her resolve to extricate herself and her child from the violence of the boy's father. As soon as the father was back in the picture, 3-year-old Tom resumed wetting himself at child care. He withdrew from any rambunctious play. Seeming to interpret other children's enthusiastic overtures as aggressive acts, he adopts an affectless stare, all the while flailing his arms as if they were unattached to his otherwise motionless little body. Separations from his mother are becoming increasingly difficult.

> After many meetings with the consultant, Tom's mother talked about their situation. She tearfully told a story of intermittent explosions punctuated by brief separations. The mother's "confession," as she called it, came after the consultant recited a particularly poignant account of Tom's behavior at child care. The consultant concluded her description with an interpretation

of Tom's internal experience. She gently suggested that Tom sometimes looked like "he had seen a ghost." Even though there was no real danger in the school situation, Tom seemed terrified.

The connection between the family's situation and Tom's behavior was immediately evident to both his mother and the consultant. Mom desperately wanted to make things different for her little boy. She was utterly helpless to imagine how. The consultant met more with Tom's mother. She attended to the family's safety and found referrals for mother and child. In the midst of this broader effort, the consultant was encouraging Mom to talk to Tom's providers. The consultant knew it was unlikely that Mom could actively protect Tom when she was not yet able to protect herself. Equally aware of the mother's deep devotion to Tom, the consultant suggested that talking with Tom's caregivers was a first step in providing safety for her son. The consultant added that until Mom was in a position to provide Tom the security she hoped to offer, the caregivers could supply some solace and stability. However, as they were currently unaware of the violence and unpredictability that characterized Tom's life, the caregivers weren't accurately perceiving or empathically responding to his needs.

Still, Mom could not bring herself to face Tom's providers. She gave the consultant permission to talk with them. The permission was, however, provisional. Speaking specifically about the domestic violence was prohibited. The consultant felt constrained, yet she did not want to replicate the mother's experience of helplessness, so she posited palatable and protective ways of talking with Tom's caregivers. She wondered if she could convey, "Tom's family was going through a very rough time that made it impossible for Mom to make home life as secure and predictable as she wanted." Mom agreed to the consultant sharing this abridged account of their lives. The consultant returned to talk with the providers, confident that by conveying the essence of his experience she could evoke the empathy and enlist the support of Tom's teachers.

Persuading a parent or provider to divulge information they perceive as damning or controversial requires sensitivity and skill. Strictly adhering to the possessor's privacy is paramount. Promising confidentiality is paired with the conviction that constructing meaning is contingent on disclosure. By extracting elements essential to the child's experience, the consultant conveys that this is the relevant information.

Distillation is beneficial even when full disclosure is granted. Communicating extensive or extraneous information can confuse or unnecessarily burden the recipient. Hearing in excruciating detail about a family's agony creates a sense of responsibility in providers to rectify circumstances beyond their control and outside their professional purview. Similarly, parents should be spared the intricacies of a program's pressures and organizational foibles if they do not directly pertain to their child's situation. Whether acting as a conduit or encouraging direct exchange, the consultant draws a circle around the child, deliberately marking this as the crucial realm of discourse. In doing so, the purpose of exchange becomes evident to all the participants.

Co-Creating the Meaning of Behavior

Using the information drawn from her observations and from the adults caring for the child, the consultant begins formulating hypotheses about the meaning of the child's behavior. The providers and the parents are engaged in developing these theories with her. Information that a caregiver is uniquely able to provide regarding the experience of being with a particular child represents an invaluable contribution to the project of deciphering the child's experience. In order for the adult's experiences of a child to contribute to co-creating meaning, a set of assumptions must be shared. The basic assumption informing the consultant's questioning is that *all behavior has meaning*. Her questions ask not only for a description of the child's actions but also for a hypothesis about the meaning. To this end, the consultant might wonder about changes in a child's home life when he is suddenly unable to separate from his parents, or the consultant might inquire as to a provider's notion of why any close peer contact evokes an outburst.

Questions like these convey the consultant's view that, although all behavior is meaningful, the causes for and meaning of behavior, even the same behavior, in different children are myriad. The task is to decipher and understand the behavior as an idiosyncratic expression of this child. The meaning is not found in the behavior itself but rather is formed and understood in the relationships in which the child is engaged. Implicit in all conversations is the assumption that children's behavior has meaning, and there is a steadfast effort at broadening the possibilities as to what these meanings may be.

Framework for Understanding Behavior

Expansive consideration of contributors to a child's behavior relies on an internalized repertoire of possibilities. In order to convey it, the consultant must possess this knowledge. This is where grounding in the vicissitudes of development—ranging from the expectable to the atypical—is essential. An appreciation of the transactional nature of development adds to a nuanced perspective.

The consultant fits what she has learned about a child into categories of possible cause. Although no human behavior has a single or pure origin, determinates are identifiable. By no means exhaustive, a few common headings under which meaning might be made are offered. The rubrics are broad and the explanations cursory, but they build on an adaptable framework for understanding children's behavior first proposed by child development specialist James Hymes (1952) more than half a century ago. Although there are many more and all are interdependent, contributory categories are outlined below. Explanations are presented from the least to the most complex. Examples of behaviors attributable to each are included.

I. Developmental Stage—as a Cause for Behavior

In each domain, development progresses in a somewhat predictable pattern. Characteristic behaviors mark a child's passage along these trajectories. Accompanying behaviors represent practicing of the phase's essential tasks. Mastery is not the exclusive aim of the child's behaviors. Repetition and reworking actually propel development. These rehearsing behaviors are known to most child-care and mental health professionals. In the physical domain, rolling over is followed by sitting, and creeping proceeds crawling, which gives way to walking. The path is usually uniform, and no one questions that an infant spends an abundant amount of energy and time at each task in order to move on to the next. Extensive study of child development and experience with children of like ages informs expectations in all domains. Therefore, behaviors reflecting practicing are not usually puzzling to child-care providers. Few expect that proficient running will immediately follow an infant's first step.

However, behaviors associated with the social–emotional sphere are often an exception. These behaviors require responsiveness, but it is more likely that providers find them frustrating because they are unaware of their crucial contribution to development. The following example illustrates a caregiver's conundrum when faced with behavior, the purpose of which eludes her.

Example

Rebecca is at her wit's end with 8-month-old Alejandro. Recently, he started sending every item she places on his tray over the high chair's edge. Following its descent, he beckons Rebecca to retrieve the spoon, cracker, or carrot as soon as it reaches its destination. He beams with delight when she replaces them, only to send them careening off again.

Baffled by this behavior, she reports it and her frustration to the consultant. After asking several questions about Alejandro's response to disappearances of other kinds, the consultant feels certain his behavior is a way of practicing object permanence. Explaining the concept as a baby's attempt to learn that things—and even more importantly, people—exist when out of sight calms Rebecca's upset. A hazy memory from her development class resurfaces. However, she wouldn't have made the connection without the consultant's help. Convinced through their conversation that Alejandro's behavior is meaningful and necessary to his development, she allows it to continue. In subsequent conversations, she and the consultant expand the opportunities for practicing. Rebecca puts out the canister in which multishaped blocks can be said good-bye to and retrieved. Playing peek-a-boo becomes the dyad's favored interaction.

II. Individual Differences—as a Cause for Behavior

Every child enters the world uniquely themselves. Whether exactly whom we hoped for or not at all who we expected, an infant's individual differences affect what he experiences and how he is experienced. Sounds that soothe one baby unnerve another. Being securely swaddled is the only way for one infant to organize, whereas another strains at the restraint until his upset is the only thing he can attend to.

Reciprocally, infants' idiosyncratic reactions cause parallel particularities in those who care for them. A baby who finds his caregiver's every action to be a delight beams his approval. Likely the provider is pleased with her perfection and with the recipient for making her feel this way. When the same interactions startle rather then soothe another of her charges, she is dismayed. Critique of her caregiving lessens her confidence. Consequently, this child is interacted with less and less favored.

The array of individual differences is as plentiful as the babies who possess them. Some are subtle; others, glaring. They are categorized for descriptive convenience. Temperamental types are partitioned. Congenital, health, or developmental conditions are labeled and diagnosed. Regulatory capacities are compartmentalized. Sensory reactivity and processing is assessed in discreet modalities, and responses in each are gauged by where they fall between the hypo- and hyper-

poles of the spectrum. Knowledge of these conceptualizations of constitutional contributors to behavior is useful.

Determining if individual differences account for behavior requires combining theoretical knowledge with retrospective research. Although often apparent early on, innate factors change form over time. A hunch that behavior is organically based is confirmed by identifying historical antecedents. Therefore, an infant's earliest caregivers, usually parents, are key informants. Tracing the origins of current expressions relies on information they alone possess. Parents can validate a hypothesis only as they are able or assisted in linking current behavior to a child's earlier modes of expression.

Example

Kyle is holed up in the classroom's quiet corner when the consultant arrives to observe him. His teacher, Tanya, has to point him out as he is completely hidden in a hive of large pillows. Tanya tells the consultant that he constructed the nest when she had to exclude him from circle time "again."

Any group gathering is difficult for Kyle, but the percussive instruments played today sent him into orbit. He crashed into other children, unable to follow his peers in the musical procession. His screeching drowned out the teacher's instruction and dwarfed the loudest drumbeat.

Kyle's wild rendition is hard to envision as he now calmly combs the pages of a book he buried with him in his hideout. He stays occupied and organized until the bell signaling clean-up time is sounded. Flinging books from his bunker, Kyle pops out like a Jack-in-the-box as the activity around him increases. As if at the eye of the storm, he stands mesmerized. His body visibly vibrating, Kyle vigorously chews the sleeve of his shirt.

On the basis of this observation and the providers' description of Kyle, the consultant constructs a theory about his behavior. Her tentative hypothesis is confirmed by talking with Kyle's parents. At first, the picture Tanya and the consultant present puzzles them. As an only child, Kyle is rarely around other children except at child care. His home life resembles the hushed area he constructed for himself at school as his parents prefer placidity and privacy. They describe their lifestyle as "laid back but orderly."

Given that home differs dramatically in the quantity and quality of stimulation, the consultant asks about occasions that imitate the school environment. She also inquires about Kyle's responses in infancy.

Letting everyone in on her hypothesis, she prefaces her questions by explaining that Kyle seems challenged by the hustle and bustle of group care, especially the decibel level. Such sensitivities are often part of a person from birth, hence, her asking about him as a baby. Connections come to mind. Kyle has always come unglued in a crowd. Loud noises were so startling that throughout infancy his parents kept him in a cap and swaddled in several blankets. The buffer not only kept out unwanted sounds but also seemed to help him stay organized and alert.

The retrospective reconstruction of Kyle's experience confirmed the consultant's hypothesis and helped everyone make sense of his current behavior. In retreating to a peaceful place and cocooning himself in pillows, Kyle was replicating the adaptations that his parents made early on to his sensory sensitivities. As a 4-year-old, Kyle's reactions and his accommodations looked different. The consultant's questions and theory provided his parents and teacher a way of linking his past and present responses, thereby uncovering the origin of his behaviors in child care.

III. The Child-Care Environment—as a Cause for Behavior

A program's physical space, organization, activities, routines, and relationships contribute to children's behavior. Determining the exact influence of environmental factors is done partially through a process of elimination. Behavior that is not expressly attributable to the previously described causes (developmental stage and individual differences) may be accounted for by environmental contributors. Less exclusively, the setting can exacerbate behaviors that reflect developmental or idiosyncratic forces.

Although every child interacts uniquely with his or her environment, similar responses among many children in a group provide an important clue. Like behavior tells us the group is reacting to a specific condition in the setting. Reciprocally, adjusting the causative agent will immediately ameliorate the troubling behavior in all who were adversely affected.

Whether an accurate assessment or a hopeful illusion, child-care providers often attempt to explain behavior as an outgrowth of the environment. They hope to infer causality to a situation over which they have control. Therefore, providers leap to structural solutions. A child who is often inattentive and disinterested in a toddler room's curriculum is prematurely placed in a preschool class. Similarly, furniture is rearranged and activities adapted in an attempt to quell group chaos. Adaptations undertaken because they are possible do not ensure accuracy as to the cause or success in alleviating the behaviors that brought them about.

In their search for environmental contributors, providers may overlook themselves. Teachers' behavior is an important aspect of the child-care environment.

Example

Lamenting the lack of interest her near 5-year-olds group shows in circle time, Grace asks for the consultant's assistance. Together they ponder possible contributors to the conundrum. The preschool teacher speculates that "spring fever" is the cause as it is May and many children will soon leave for kindergarten. As the consultant pursues Grace's theory, they both become less convinced of its accuracy.

Although the spiraling into silliness that brings circle time to an abrupt end on most days could support Grace's notion, similar behavior is rarely displayed in other parts of the day. Art projects are engaged in with vigor. Other small group activities capture rapt attention.

With this new information, the consultant concentrates on the conditions that exist exclusively in circle time. She confines her conversations with Grace to discussion about characteristics of this routine. Wondering together reveals several recent adaptations. Feeling mounting pressure to prepare children for the transition to "school," Grace extended the length of circle time to incorporate lessons she hopes will accelerate academic achievement. Familiar songs that had always been accompanied with movement were replaced by sit-in-place recitations of the day's weather conditions, roll call, and letter recognition. Hand raising was now expected when previously spontaneous interaction had been encouraged. The perceived necessity of this transformation momentarily blinded this usually perceptive teacher to the impact of the shift on the children's behavior. The removed and less impassioned eye of the consultant helped Grace regain perspective. As the teacher reconciled her wish to prepare with the children's capacities and readiness, circle time became manageable. The immediate improvement in children's behavior signaled that the cause had been correctly identified.

IV. The Home Environment—as a Cause for Behavior

Like the child-care environment, happenings in the home contribute to children's behavior. Pervasive environmental influences, such as culture and ways of relating, will be discussed in subsequent sections. Here we consider specific incidences and events. Environmental occurrences range from mundane to major milestones to devastating disruptions (e.g., grandparents visit; shifts in sleeping arrangements are negotiated; parents gain or lose jobs; siblings are born; someone in the family is sick or dies). The impact in small ripples or waves will be expressed in children's behavior. Experience in one context, regardless of intensity or predictability can transform a child's feelings, expectations, and responses in other venues. Effects are evidenced in child care.

When the child-care provider–parent relationship is strong and an atmosphere of exchange exists, happenings in the home are usually shared. However, the absence of these conditions, as well as other factors, precludes access to information that would assist providers in making sense of a child's behavior. Lack of disclosure may be purposeful or unintentional. A slight change in routine goes unnoticed by parents and yet shakes the security of a sensitive infant. Parents cannot alert the child's providers to a swerve they did not register. Likewise, a known occurrence may not be acknowledged because the family anticipates an unfavorable or critical response.

Without information, for whatever reason, providers must rely on what they witness in the child's behavior to unravel the mystery of its meaning. Sudden change in a child's behavior is the most likely indicator that the cause is environmental. Rapid regression or uncharacteristic expressions suggest an external trigger. All surroundings should be examined. Eliminating any ready explanation in the child-care environment, the familial surround is turned to for clues.

Parents are essential informants in the discovery process. Their assistance is encouraged only as its relevance is made clear and fears about disclosure are relieved. The providers and consultant pave the way by conveying nonjudgmental interest in understanding and assisting the child.

Example

Sergio's father often brings him to school, but for the past week this is the exclusive arrangement. His arrival and his father's departure are increasingly wrenching events. The toddler clings and wails plaintively as Dad tries to placate and peel Sergio from him. The handoff to his adored primary caregiver, Adelina, offers little solace. Sergio remains irritable even though he is carried and caressed for most of the morning. Adelina tries to no avail to interest the boy in his favorite toys. By midday, Sergio seems almost himself. He ventures from his caregiver to engage in play. However, he returns regularly for refueling and keeps a watchful eye on Adelina.

At pick-up time, Adelina describes Sergio's distress and her eventually effective attempts to soothe it, to his father. She wonders if Sergio is coming down with something and asks the father if he has noticed the child's uncharacteristic difficulty at separations and his increased fussiness. While mumbling agreement, the father offers no explanation. He seems preoccupied and skittish. The pair departs quickly, leaving Sergio's bottle and jacket behind.

The next week brings bigger concerns. In addition to distress, Sergio now refuses food and is rarely able to nap. Adelina's growing worry prompts a call to the consultant. Hearing about the sudden and dramatic shift in both Sergio and his father's behavior, the consultant posits a possibility. "The deterioration you describe sounds so swift, it makes me wonder if there has been a big change in the family's life?" The question supports Adelina's intuition. Specifically, she suspects the dyad's difficulties are somehow related to Sergio's mother, who has not been seen at the center for weeks now. Adelina wants to inquire about Mom's whereabouts because she wants to help Sergio, but the father's increasing avoidance makes her apprehensive. She doesn't want to overstep her role or invade the family's privacy.

Knowing the trust and mutual respect that preceded this difficult patch in the provider–parent relationship, the consultant encourages Adelina to talk with Sergio's father in much the same way she spoke to her. The consultant reiterates Adelina's intention—she is concerned about Sergio and his father, and she cares deeply about their well-being. Her wish is to offer support. She might be better able to address Sergio's distress if she had a sense of what was contributing to it, but she doesn't want Dad to feel that she is prying into personal matters.

By capturing and reflecting Adelina's sentiments, the consultant helps her recognize the compassion they carry. Talking with Sergio's father feels less daunting. The spirit of the caregiver's message relieves Dad's apprehension. He tells Adelina of his wife's return to their native country to care for her dying mother. The telling, like the journey itself, felt treacherous because the family is undocumented. Assured that Adelina's concern is the family's well-being, not their legal status in this county, the adults could turn their attention to helping Sergio cope with the separation from his mother.

Unburdened of the need to hide his wife's absence, Sergio's father eagerly responds to Adelina's suggestion that a picture of Mom and a scent-laden sweater be brought to child care. Adelina uses herself and these items as prompts for Sergio's sustained security. Snuggled in his mother's wrap, Adelina sings to Sergio in Spanish the lullabies his mother puts him to sleep with each night. Gazing at the picture affixed to his crib, Sergio's eyes shut slowly. He and his caregiver rest more peacefully in the space of understanding and being understood.

V. Culture—as a Cause for Behavior

Every aspect of human existence is touched and altered by culture. From birth, babies are viewed and come to view who they are through the filter of their family's culture. Given the expanse of culture's influence, we could safely say that all behavior bears its mark.

Behaviors reflecting cultural values and beliefs are challenged or challenging when they rub up against alternate expectations and interpretations. At this interface a child's behavior may be puzzling to a provider who looks through a distinct lens. As a rule, our worldview is so deeply ingrained that we mistake it for reality. Unexamined ethnocentrism can be an obstacle to accurately interpreting the meaning of another's actions. When these misperceptions are accompanied by judgment, the problem is compounded. Mislabeling combined with devaluing is especially dangerous for young children.

Children are caught in an untenable conflict when important adults in their lives value different ways of behaving. A child's culture encourages dependency, whereas autonomy is rewarded at child care. Averting one's gaze signals respect at home but is admonished at school. None of these practices are inherently honorable or disdainful. However, when they are weighted in a particular direction, a child experiences himself as displeasing to an essential adult. Young children rely on the approval of their parents and their child-care providers. Each one's opinion of him matters. Both groups' sense of the rightness or wrongness of his behavior influences not only how we will act but, more importantly, how he feels about himself for behaving in a certain manner. Caught between competing adult values, children feel they must choose. Children cannot afford losing the approval, love, or support of either faction.

Ascribing value to customary ways of expressing oneself is not in and of itself problematic. No child-care program can perfectly replicate the cultural practices of each of its constituents, especially when a broad multicultural mix of providers, parents, and children is represented, nor must child care abandon its "culture" in favor of instilling alternate ideals. When expectations are offered without suggesting that they are the only or right way, children compartmentalize and internalize a range of acceptable ways of behaving. Preschool-age children quickly come to know the tone of voice that accompanies indoor versus outside activities. Grandparents often allow a wider behavioral berth than Mom and Dad. Similarly, when value is extracted from varying cultural practices, children respond according to the prescribed expectations. The benefit and beauty of different cultural customs is retained. Concomitantly, the child is pleasing to, and pleased by his behavior with, all of the important adults in his life.

Example

Having recently fled their ravaged war-torn village in the Sudan, Shihar and her husband needed to find work. Reluctantly, they placed 13-month-old Waleed in child care. Carefully unwrapping the infant from the reams of cloth that attached him to her back, Shihar positioned him each morning on the floor in a corner of the infant room, a spot from which he rarely moved. Carried to a high chair and strapped in, Waleed became more animated. He smiled and babbled at the caregivers who placed chunks of cheese and precisely cut apple slices on the tray. Inspecting the offerings with his eyes, Waleed ate only what was fed to him.

Soon his lack of initiation brought his providers perplexed attention. Confusion was eclipsed by concern as Waleed's statuesque stance and refusal to feed himself continued. Speaking to their consultant about their worries, she noted a tinge of frustration in the providers' description of this child's behavior. Feeding and carrying Waleed took extra time, of which they had little to spare. Speculating that overprotective pampering accounted for Waleed's dependency, the providers were becoming less enamored of his parents and equally unenthusiastic about the baby.

Unable to imagine an alternate explanation for what the providers labeled "spoiled," the consultant wondered if she might involve Waleed's parents in the investigation. Baffled by both the caregivers' concern and their expectations of Waleed, Shihar offered an explanation. Protection was, as the caregivers suspected, this mother's motivation, but it was not excessive or for the purpose of pampering. Her baby was discouraged from putting food or any other object in his mouth. Given the contaminated water and often rancid foodstuffs in their native area, the prohibition prevented disease or death. Similarly, letting a toddler roam unattached to an adult's body invited disaster. Surprise enemy ambushes left little time to corral a crawler who strayed too far. Even before the threat of attack necessitated this practice, Shihar's culture encouraged the constant carrying of children under the age of 3. Shihar explained that fire pits were used to cook. Little ones could be severely burned.

Once shared, Shihar's information shifted the providers' views of her and Waleed. A dialogue between the parents and providers helped each group to develop appreciation for the others' perspectives and practices. As trust in the providers' intentions and their ability to keep Waleed safe expanded, so did his willingness to explore. Freed of his mother's fear and his providers' frustration, Waleed sensed security in being carried at home and crawling at child care. Being fed felt good, and it was good to feed himself.

VI. Unmet Social and Emotional Needs as a Cause for Behavior

Human beings share a set of basic needs. In addition to physical requirements, we all have fundamental emotional and social needs. Babies are social beings, who from the beginning are able to elicit in their caregivers a powerful motivation to provide protection and care. Infants are utterly dependent on adults to reciprocate. Reciprocity, mutuality, safety, and predictability must be consistent features of a child's interpersonal world if he is to develop trust, security, and a sense of efficacy.

When these needs are not routinely recognized, a child's sense of self and view of the world is shaped by what's lacking. Unfulfilled, the need intensifies. The child is driven to try to satisfy the growing hunger. These attempts are often witnessed in disturbing or disturbed behaviors. The outward expression rarely reveals the underlying need. A child who has not been adequately protected—or worse yet, repeatedly hurt—is unlikely to be able to ask for, or in any way directly demonstrate his yearning for, safety. The distortion, his inability to "ask," is a result of his experience of not having the need met. A child can't expect what has never been received. Expectations determine perception. We interpret the present through the lens of expectations created from cumulative past experiences to the point of perceiving what we expect to receive.

The child who has known far too little security looks at the world through a lens that refracts only danger. The world is not a safe place about which one can be curious or eagerly explore. Adults are cast with the same suspicious glare. They cannot be counted on to care or turned to for help. The child's sense of self is the flip side of this negative filter. If the world and people in it are dangerous, he must rely on himself. Self-protection comes in few forms for young children. You can completely withdraw, hoping through disappearance to avoid the world's harshness, or start swinging at the slightest threat, attempting to proactively prevent the inevitable assaults the world has thus far offered. Either way, the need is rarely realized.

Although unsuccessful and based on misperceptions, the behavior persists. These troubling expressions abate as the social–emotional need is satisfied. This is possible only in the context of a reparative adult relationship in which the underlying message is understood and the child's negative expectations are consistently violated through actions that provide protection and security. The child whose behaviors belie a pressing need is often the most difficult for providers to understand and empathize with; yet this is the child most in need of such an attuned relationship.

Example

After just a few months in child care, Cole is, from his providers' reports, doing better. The consultant comes to observe the improvement. She has, since shortly after his enrollment in the center, been involved in the effort to understand and assist him. Cole is the first to notice her arrival. He proceeds to point out the rules and routines he now clings to as guideposts of predictability. The verbal repertoire of this 2-year-old is limited, but he gets his point across. Pulling at the consultant's foot and pointing to the nearby cubbies, he conveys that visitors must remove their shoes. Patting a cushioned bench, he instructs her to have a seat. With the consultant properly situated, Cole crosses the room. Movement from the assigned spot is reprimanded with a forceful reminder. Cole's behavior seems to say, "If everything stays just so, I might too."

Sharing this interpretation with his providers, the consultant hears numerous confirming examples of Cole's reactions to change. Already this morning, he has had two explosive outbursts; the first was in response to finding that a favored toy was not in its usual spot. When shown it still existed, he could not be calmed. He now clutches the object under his arm, carrying but not playing with it. A child who brushes by is pushed to the ground. Cole screams, "No mine," protecting a possession from someone who has expressed no interest in it.

The other earlier incident was prompted by a change in paper products. The cartoon characters parading around the periphery of the morning juice cups were unfamiliar. This deviation sent Cole into spasms of inconsolable upset. The litany of infractions that could jostle Cole's fragile emotional equilibrium was long. His naptime bedding was washed on the weekend as its disappearance during the week was intolerable. Despite the provider's preparing him for their breaks, he batted and bit them at both departure and return. Given the inherent unpredictability of other toddlers, his peers were frequent targets. While unable to play or take pleasure in other's activities, Cole kept vigilant watch over everyone. Rarely could he get them to cooperate by staying put as the consultant had. Despite Cole's growing certainty in child care, moment-to-moment uncertainty shook him.

Cole's need for predictability and protection made sense to all who knew his early experience. Removed in early infancy from parents whose mental illness, in unfortunate combination with substance abuse, severely limited their ability to care for him, Cole was in his third foster-care placement. He had known little of safety or sameness in his short life. His behavior in child care bespoke attempts to garner both, albeit unsuccessfully. Tentative trust in his child-care providers accounted for his incremental improvement, but as yet the reservoir of alternate experience was shallow. He couldn't expect adults, even completely caring ones, to provide emotional stability. Until convinced otherwise, he must fend for himself in the ways available to a 2-year-old in a world he sees as unstable and scary.

Investigation informed by this framework propels the process of deciphering meaning. The goal is two-tiered. Determining contributors to a particular child's behavior is the explicit and immediate aim. Underlying this intent is the broader effort of encouraging providers to expansively employ the framework and the assumptions upon which it rests.

Rather than providing already assembled conclusions, the consultant includes providers in the process of co-creating meaning. Inclusion occurs as providers are asked to speculate about and develop their own hypotheses. Concomitantly, when the consultant offers a formulation, it is coupled with explanation as to how she arrived at a conclusion. The dynamic process serves an educative as well as a specific purpose. Caregivers incorporate the framework for understanding behavior. Once internalized, they can employ and generalize this template to situations beyond that of a child who is the current focus of consultation.

Case Example

As we revisit Justin, the consultant is constructing a sphere of consideration with his providers. She offers purposely selected segments of her conversations with his grandmother. In doing so, she promotes reciprocal understanding among all concerned with Justin's welfare. Simultaneously, she and the providers take to the path of co-creating meaning. Progress is initially threatened by Justin's increasing distress and the discouragement this causes his providers.

> Between the consultant's observations and her meetings with Mrs. Jones, she was meeting with the child-care staff. During this time, Justin's difficulties were escalating. In turn, the staff's frustration and helplessness increased. At the next staff meeting, the consultant is faced with the provider's urgency for answers. As the group sits around a tiny table among sleeping children, one of the providers, Tometrius, announces, "I hope by now you've figured out what to do with him. If something doesn't change soon, I don't think Justin can stay here. Other kids are getting hurt, their parents are constantly complaining, and we are exhausted."

> Knowing that the providers' feelings figure prominently in their willingness to persevere, the consultant acknowledges the growing concern. She does not try to convince the caregivers to keep Justin. Instead, she explores the limits of their capacity to continue. She asks about what would have to change and how immediately it would have to be different. In doing so, she places decision making back where it belongs, with the child-care program. Then, the consultant reminds staff that they, not she, are the agents of change: "I wish it were as easy as me giving the answer. If it were simple, we'd have figured it out already. I have some new ideas to offer based on my recent

observations and meetings with Mrs. Jones. But it may feel like too little, too late. You're the ones who have to put ideas into actions, so you've got the harder job here. Given how trying the past month has been, is there any room left to consider continuing?"

Beleaguered but dedicated, the staff agrees to entertain the new information. Having Mrs. Jones' permission, the consultant adds Justin's history and her observations to the conversation. Beginning with anecdotes from her observations, she reminds the providers of behavior they collectively witnessed. Encountering a stranger, Justin cowered. While reminiscent of his early days at the center, withdrawal was now an aberration. It was agreed that Justin's response could be attributed to fear of the unfamiliar. Seeing Justin's reaction as responsive to specific circumstances, the providers could entertain rather than discount these differences as meaningful information. In this context, the consultant presents the contrasting image of the boy she observed at home and school. She admits that she, like the staff, found the discrepancy hard to believe. She is quick to add that after meeting with Mrs. Jones she is less baffled. Her conversations with Mrs. Jones provide some clues.

Knowing that the providers don't see Mrs. Jones as a reliable source of information and that they question her commitment to Justin, the consultant prefaces sharing information by saying, "Like you, Mrs. Jones had given this a lot of thought. She too was confused about the differences in Justin. But together she and I came up with some possible explanations. I'm eager to hear if you think our theory makes any sense."

The consultant then speaks about Justin's experiences of abrupt separation and loss. Careful to curtail her comments so as not to burden the providers or infer blame, she speaks specifically about the effects on Justin forgoing a blow-by-blow account of his history. Striking this balance by saying, "Neither of Justin's parents is in a position to care for him right now. They each seem to be struggling just to stay afloat for themselves. Although Mrs. Jones tries to keep contact for Justin's sake, his parents' instability makes it hard. Justin's dad is in jail, and his mother is homeless right now. Also, since there were concerns about how Justin was cared for by his mother, she is not allowed to spend time with him alone. So, it's all up to Mrs. Jones. She wants Justin to know and feel he can count on his parents, but a lot gets in the way of making that happen. Logistics are part of it. She works on the weekends to make ends meet. Sometimes that keeps Justin from visiting his dad. Even when Grandma can make time, it doesn't always work out. It sounds like it's hard for Justin's mom to visit regularly."

As she spoke, the consultant registered oscillations in the emotional climate. As the group's barometer, she gave voice to the feelings floating around the room, all the while locating Justin's experience at the center of the affective storm: "As adults we might disapprove of the parents' actions or be mad at them, but we can at least understand why they can't care for Justin. He can't. I imagine he feels some horrible mix of fear, anger, and longing: fear of losing the little he has come to trust; anger, not just at Mom and Dad but probably with anybody who he feels has, or will, take away what he is clinging to; and longing for someone to make sense of his world and make it safe. You might be feeling just as jumbled: sad for Justin, angry at anyone who's contributed to his life being so complicated, upset at me for telling you, or at Mrs. Jones for taking so long to let you know."

Sensing the last sentiment struck a nerve, the consultant explains Mrs. Jones' position, "When I asked Mrs. Jones what it was like for her when Justin arrived unannounced less than a year ago at her doorstep, she described him as skittery, scared, and stubborn. I think she wanted to erase that really difficult time from memory. Who wouldn't? Recalling what it was like really helped her appreciate what you all are going through now. I also think it will help us."

Initially angered by Mrs. Jones' amnesia, the staff expresses uncertainty about the usefulness of the information. The providers' dismay with Mrs. Jones was expressed by Tometrius, "Don't get me wrong, I wouldn't wish that mess on anyone, but it doesn't excuse Mrs. Jones. It's too convenient—her forgetting he was a wreck just long enough for us to feel we'd caused all Justin's problems." A bit more empathic with Mrs. Jones, Latania is perplexed at how the information is of use to them: "Believe me, there are painful parts of my past I'd rather not remember, but what I don't get is how that's going to help us now?" The consultant makes the connection between Justin's past experiences and his present behavior.

The consultant initially focuses on Justin's entry into child care, given the tenor of interstaff and parent–staff relationships at the time. None of the adults had been able to support each other. Therefore, Justin was left to fend for himself in an unfamiliar situation. His initial response was to withdraw. The consultant suggests that his timidity was likely out of terror. Justin then started to assert himself through aggression. This progression was reminiscent of what Mrs. Jones had seen when Justin came into her care. It was also mirrored in the microcosm of the consultant's observations.

As these issues were discussed in several subsequent consultation meetings, the caregivers felt less responsible for causing the behavior. Freed from guilt and their conflict with Mrs. Jones, their empathy for Justin increased. The staff could now consider the meaning of the behavior that previously puzzled and infuriated them. The consultant offered connections between Justin's history of separations and unpredictability and his behavior at child care. She fastened Justin's past to the present with concrete examples, making statements like, "Justin has had so many unexplained losses in his life. I wonder if he worries that letting go of anything means it will be gone forever. I'm thinking about how he clings to Grandma in the morning and to you, Sue, when you put him down for nap. I'm realizing his worry is sort of confirmed. Once he says good-bye to Grandma, she's gone for the day. And Sue, isn't it true that your shift ends at 2:00 p.m.? So you're not here when he wakes up. A day seems short to us, but I bet it feels like an eternity to a little one who has had so much disappear. I can see why he's holding on for dear life to two people he's come to trust will be there for him. I bet it's not easy to see his screaming at naptime as a sign of how important you are to him, but I think it's his only way right now of letting us know how much he relies on you."

About smaller shifts, the consultant remarks, "I know you want to rotate the activities so children have choices. I can't help but wonder if the end of the transportation theme contributed to Justin's tantrum today. You were telling me last week he had, for the first time, settled into play. He really liked that train set you had out. He got here today, and it was gone. I know other children benefit from variety. Justin can't take pleasure in newness yet. It might seem like a small thing, but I think for Justin change is only associated with loss."

The caregivers came to see transitions as anxiety-producing reminders of loss. The link to major transitions such as drop-off and naptime was immediately apparent. The consultant highlighted the ways in which small shifts, like changes in the routine or where a toy was placed, also aroused anxiety. Although harder to empathize with or tolerate, the meaning of Justin's aggressive behavior was also becoming comprehensible. The consultant helped the providers to see the world through Justin's lens of negative expectations. Given his experiences of sudden loss and possible abuse, he likely saw others as a threat. His aggressive outbursts were his way of protecting himself from danger. Justin's lashing out when he was approached by peers was seen as an attempt to defend against being hurt or having objects or ideas taken from him.

This segment of Justin's case started shakily. The providers threatened to expel him. They pressed the consultant for immediate answers and simple solutions. Fortunately, the consultant avoided this frequently laid trap. Had she been less sure of her stance, she would have quickly moved to offer "expert" advice. Her suggestions, regardless of objective accuracy, would have been ill-fated.

Faced with pressure to "tell providers what to do," the consultant reminds herself and them that making meaning of a child's behavior is not simple but necessary. Instead of acting, the consultant empathizes with the providers' helplessness and anger. If she does away with these feelings, she imagines the source, Justin, will not have to be.

Having successfully traversed the treacherous terrain of Justin's possible expulsion, the consultant delicately discloses Justin's history. She carefully chooses not only when but what she will share from her conversations with Mrs. Jones. Premised on the permission she was granted, the consultant balances protecting the participants with the need to say enough. Too fulsome an accounting would have run the risk of burdening the providers with a responsibility to cure ills that they had not caused and for which they could not completely compensate. Alternately, concentrating on parental limitations and foibles could have bogged the process down in finger pointing. The consultant arduously avoids affixing blame.

Finding fault is not the purpose. Offering possible explanations for Justin's current behavior is. The consultant begins to weave the strands of Justin's experience into a cohesive explanation, linking meaning and causation to current behavior. The consultant connects Justin's presentation in child care to persisting unmet emotional needs. She is aware of bringing providers along in the construction. Implicit in the consultant's conversations with staff was her assumption that Justin's behavior had meaning. She steadfastly worked at identifying the meaning. All along she encourages the providers' internalization of a framework for assessing and understanding the multiple contributors to behavior in hopes that one day they will make it their own. While focusing on Justin and the specifics of his experience, the consultant's agenda with caregivers extends beyond this case. Incorporating the assumptions that underlie her process for making meaning is her broader goal.

When caregivers are proceeding from these assumptions, they are able to make use of their own internal responses to a child in the service of forming hypotheses about the way the child feels the world and himself to be. From here they are in an excellent position to assist him in feeling less bewildered and more trusting in the world. Freeing providers from misconceptions and helping them to consider that *all behavior has meaning*, are necessary precursors to action.

Summary

Usually providers and parents can eloquently describe a child's behavior. Description proceeds but is not synonymous with understanding. Establishing similarities or differences between what is seen and uncovering the contributors to and meaning of behavior propel the process. The consultant guides the discovery. First, she sets out to open clogged channels of communication between providers and parents if obstacles exist. While respecting the privacy of each participant, the consultant gently encourages direct exchange as she is aware that information about a child is useful only as it shared and mutually accepted as accurate.

While building bridges of direct dialogue, the consultant is communicating through a stance of curiosity her assumption that all behavior is meaningful. She asks the other adults to join her in elaborating on the possible causes for and ways of interpreting behavior. Throughout the journey of generating hypotheses the consultant contributes her expertise in the form of knowledge about the vicissitudes of development, both typical and extraordinary. Synthesizing everyone's information and knowledge is the consultant's ultimate aim in this phase of consultation.

Reference

Hymes, J. (1952). *Understanding your child.* Old Tappan, NJ: Prentice-Hall.

Chapter 9

Translating Meaning Into Responsive Action—Within and Alongside the Child-Care Setting

Case consultation culminates in translating understanding into action. Moving from accurately interpreting meaning to responsiveness is an organic process. Shifts in the providers' relationships with a child are often an outgrowth of increased awareness of and empathy for a child whose actions are compatible with the underlying causes uncovered in the previous stages of consultation. The consultant supports these naturally occurring amendments. When these shifts in relationships are not automatic, the consultant intercedes and explores the impediments to attunement.

At the providers' request and as obstacles erode, the consultant joins in the construction of interventions. She offers ideas and inserts suggestions aimed at ameliorating the child's difficulties and the providers' struggles. Aware of her place in the implementation of any intervention, the consultant is careful not to prescribe or assume. She again employs the "wondering" stance and supports the providers (and parents) as the ultimate agents of change.

Once meaning is cooperatively constructed, a shared perspective established, and action to ameliorate a child's distress is underway, case consultation typically concludes. However, consultation can be extended when a child's needs exceed this effort and the confines of the child-care setting. The consultant's role expands to referral source and advocate.

Translating Understanding of a Child's Behavior Into Responsive Action

Moving from understanding to action is the final, and sometimes imperceptible, activity of case consultation. As a child's behavior becomes more comprehensible, caregivers are better able to respond empathically. Their confidence about the potentially positive influence of their relationship with the child also increases. Understanding the meaning of behavior and feeling that her relationship can be an agent of change often shifts the provider's way of being with a child. A relational shift promoted by increased empathy and accurate appraisal of the factors contributing to a child's distress is the central ameliorative component—the empathic exchange with an attentive caregiver improves a child's ability to trust relationships and mediate experience. The expanded or altered perspective is often a sufficient catalyst for corollary changes in the child.

As providers recognize the centrality of their relationships with children, their interest in considering new ways of interacting with a child is heightened. In this context, the caregivers can usefully incorporate the consultant's suggestions and specific expertise. Responsive actions are, like all other aspects of the consultative process, constructed collaboratively.

Providers are encouraged to communicate their understanding of the meaning of the child's behavior, first to the consultant and then to the child directly. If needed, the consultant helps providers voice their ideas. She also assists providers in finding appropriate words or ways to express themselves to the child. The consultant does this by listening carefully to the providers' responses to the questions she poses regarding the developing hypothesis. She synthesizes the providers' speculations as to the meaning of behavior. For instance, in the course of consultative conversations about a child with auditory sensitivities, the consultant integrates and translates what she is hearing by saying, "You've identified a consistent pattern. It's really difficult for Theo to stay focused if the group is doing anything loud. When it's really noisy, he becomes the whirling dervish you describe. Is that an accurate interpretation?"

The consultant's skill in translating extends beyond the providers. She helps them not only to articulate their hypothesis but also to communicate in a manner the child will understand. Young children can understand and benefit from inclusion in the process of generating notions about the meaning of their behavior.

Obviously, the ways in which a child participates in this process is distinct from the adults and dependent on his or her developmental capabilities. The child confers validity on the hypothesis the adults develop. The accuracy of the interpretations will be reflected in the child's responses. Here again, our attention is directed to the child's behavior and what it is telling us.

The consultant communicates her belief in the value of the child's participation in two ways. She gives voice to the child's experience. She also encourages providers to involve the child in their evolving understanding of him. Respectively, these two vehicles for promoting the child's inclusion take the form of speaking *for the child* and helping providers speak *to the child* (nonverbally as well as with words).

Returning to the previous scenario, the consultant might begin to bring the child's experience into focus by imagining how unsettling a large group must be for 4-year-old Theo, who seems to have come into the world without the mechanism that permits most of us to regulate auditory input. Speaking for Theo, the consultant says, "It's like his behavior is saying to us, 'Will you be my volume control because everything starts to sound like static and then I can't figure out what to do or where to go?'" Having provided an opening through which to view Theo's internal world, the consultant speaks to what inhabiting such a space is like.

As the consultant invites the child-care providers to venture into a child's experience and gives voice to this experience, empathy and understanding for the child increase. As the providers' empathy expands so does the interest in conveying it directly to the child. Fueled by this empathetic understanding, providers often initiate new ways of responding to a child on the basis of their already established relationship.

Acquiring or expanding one's ability to convey a deeply felt sense of a child's experience is at the heart of responsive action. A relationship imbued with such expressed understanding of another's subjective experience is the mutative factor, which the consultant is trying to nurture.

Having located the providers within Theo's internal landscape, the consultant inquires about their sense of his experience. She hears astute iterations of the ideas she and the providers developed. Providers posit their assumptions: "He must be so confused about why we get frustrated with him for not paying attention." or "Given our group size and the way sound bounces around in the room, his little insides must be jittery most of the time. No wonder he can't sit still."

Appreciating the providers' keen sense of Theo, the consultant wonders whether he is aware of their ideas about him. Incorporating what she knows about the providers' capacities and style of communication, the consultant offers ways they can share their awareness. The consultant conveys that the child will benefit from knowing that the provider sees how he experiences the world and who he feels himself to be.

Consultative discussions addressing responsive interaction are carried on over the course of many meetings. Condensing comments that would be strung out over several conversations, the consultant conveys, "Letting Theo know what you've figured out could be helpful to him. I think over time he will be better able to see you for who you are trying to be to him as he comes to trust that you genuinely understand and appreciate his struggles. After all, aren't any of us more inclined to seek out people we feel understand us? I think children are similar to adults in that way. What we have to figure out is how to get your message across. I wonder if you could notice when he begins to get overstimulated and let him know you think the big noise in the room is making his little body very excited. You probably have the best chance of being heard if you can catch him before activity is at a fevered pitch and he becomes unregulated. Gently guiding him out of the commotion and talking to him in a quieter area may make it easier for him to hear you. Offering an alternative to what he experiences as chaos will help him to stay focused, especially if you stay with him. Does that sound possible?"

The consultant translates the now mutually held understanding of the child's needs into responsive action. How she offers her ideas is as important as what she is suggesting. As illustrated by the question at the conclusion of the previous example, the consultant inquires about the feasibility and sensibleness of her suggestions. She does not shy away from offering her conceptualization as to what types of intervention or interaction might assist the child. Her suggestions are based on her understanding of the child's needs and the program's and the provider's capacities. The consultant is aware of the constraints that group care and a particular setting create.

Obstacles to Responsive Action

The consultant explores possible obstacles to the providers' responsiveness. The barriers to responsive action may reside in a particular provider, in the adult relationships, or in the program itself. A caregiver's sensitivity to a child may be blocked by an idiosyncratic intrapsychic response. A provider's past may lead her to inaccurately attribute meaning to a child's behavior. This distortion precludes emphatic responsiveness.

Cultural constructs, as well as personal histories, influence ideas about development and child-rearing practices. Typically, diverse ideas expand the ways in which meaning is made. Occasionally though, individual beliefs and cultural convictions are clung to in the face of a child exhibiting evidence to the contrary. In these instances, a provider's lens limits her ability to embrace an alternate practice or style of interaction. Differing views among staff can also interfere in constructing a consistent intervention. Discord about how a child should be treated can result in providers offering contradictory, and therefore confusing, responses. Caught in the middle of adult conflict, the child is less likely to absorb the benefits of interactions, even those attuned to his needs.

Agreement among a group of providers caring for a child does not ensure optimal attunement. Staff solidarity can keep a group of providers from adapting their interaction to the needs of a specific child in an effort to preserve group cohesiveness. Beyond staff dynamics, a program's characteristics can compromise rather than support staff in amending practices for an individual child. Aspects of a program's philosophy, the physical setting, or staffing patterns may not lend themselves to the responsive action a child requires.

The construct of group care can, in and of itself, limit a program's ability to provide optimal interactions. Children who demand moment-to-moment monitoring in order to stay regulated or to intercept aggressive outbursts tax the tolerance of a system. The very idea of accommodating an individual child's need often raises concerns among a caregiving team. Attending to the needs of the individual strikes some providers as antithetical to the purpose of group care. This is true especially when providers perceive an intervention as excessive or different from the ways children in their care are typically treated. Individually tailored treatment of a child is seen as unfair to the other children. Additionally, providers express apprehension that altering a program practice for one child will invariably cause a cascade of need in the cohort. Suggesting that a child who is unable to settle at circle time might attend better and disrupt the group less if he is offered a teacher's lap to sit on incites worries about fairness and the fear of manufacturing need in other children. Caregivers often express their concern by saying something like, "If he gets to, all the other children will want to. Then what will we do?"

Worries about what constitutes equality and fair treatment of children needs to be anticipated and addressed by the consultant. Around the often-occurring issue of fairness, a consultant could wonder whether treating everyone identically is actually synonymous with fairness. Exploring analogous adult situations is often useful. For instance, the consultant wonders if the staff members ever needed something from their director for which they wished or requested individual consideration. Then, she would inquire about what it meant to have their individual appeal responded to or not attended to. The consultant underscores that individuals in a group have different needs. Likely these idiosyncratic needs did not morph to match those of their colleagues just because the others' request was honored. Obviously, parallels between the providers and children are drawn.

Raising analogous situations to which caregivers can relate, as was done in this example, is often useful in shifting perspectives and heightening empathy. Specifically, the consultant engages caregivers in grappling with a frequently occurring dilemma in child care. Together, the consultant and providers face the struggle of balancing individual and group needs. Contemplating ways of addressing the idiosyncratic needs of a particular child, especially when the needs are extreme, arouses feelings of responsibility to the larger group.

While exploring the issues and feelings exacerbated by the constraints of caring for children in groups, consultants must genuinely appreciate the limits such circumstances place on child-care providers. Clinically trained mental health professionals typically place the parameters of their thinking around the individual child. The broad minded among us may include parents in our purview for consideration. Consulting to child care stretches these boundaries. A consultant, even when exclusively addressing concerns about an individual child, must constantly consider the context. Any advice and every suggestion are configured with the specific setting and the confines of group care in mind.

Steadfastly holding the context and having learned about the particular child-care community, the consultant formulates intervention strategies. As she offers her ideas, she also invites and is eager to be reminded of what providers feel is possible or completely impractical when she is over-enthusiastic in joining the construction of the intervention. The consultant acknowledges that, no matter how well she feels she knows a particular program, provider, or child, there may be conditions she is unaware of that make her suggestions inappropriate or undoable. Inevitably, the success of any strategy is dependent on the caregivers' genuine sense of its usefulness and their ability to enact it. Even the most brilliant recommendation is doomed to fail if the caregivers are not convinced of its merit, as they are the agents of implementation.

Case Example

The caregivers' empathy for Justin expanded in direct proportion to their appreciation of his unmet emotional needs. In the course of their continuing discussion, the staff and consultant translated their mutually agreed-upon understanding of Justin into ways of responding to his need for protection and predictability. Comings and goings were the sites for intervening and therefore the topic of several staff meetings. Changes in the in-between routines were also considered.

> Speculating that the tone for Justin's day was set by his separation from Grandma, the staff wanted to focus on the early morning transition. Now willing to include Mrs. Jones in their thinking and planning, the staff invited her to join a meeting with the consultant. The center director, Paula, also participated. Having been kept abreast of the group's efforts and surprised by the turnaround in staff sentiment toward Justin's grandma, Paula wanted to lend her supportive presence. Starting the meeting by commenting on the solidarity it represented, the consultant welcomed everyone, "Our being together speaks volumes to your commitment to Justin. He's got quite a dedicated team here. Today, we agreed to try to tackle the time of day that seems central to him and most trying to all of you—the morning good-bye. First, I wonder if we have a shared notion of why this time is the most difficult."
>
> Mrs. Jones spoke first, admitting that she was often eager to deposit Justin in child care so she could attend to her other responsibilities. She imagined Justin sensed her urgency and the preoccupation that preceded their good-bye, "My mind's already out the door before I ever set foot in here." Resonating with the rushed pace, Tometrius and Latania added that they weren't able to attend to Justin in the way they knew he needed, given the duties of diapering, breakfast, and group greeting. Sue passed. Because her shift started after Justin arrived, she could not speak to the particulars of these early morning moments. Speculating that Justin must feel a bit at sea, the consultant wondered what, if anything, the group envisioned could contribute to a calm handoff. Addressing the consultant, Mrs. Jones offered, "Since you and I've been talking, I've come to see that boy's got radar for

being left. My not being 100% there for him might make him feel like I'm gonna cut out on him like his mamma and daddy. I'd like to assure him, but sometimes I'm so tired I don't know if I'm going to make it though the day myself. He probably feels that." The providers jumped in to comfort and commiserate. Empathizing with each one's exhaustion and uncertainty, the consultant wondered if the collective sense of abandonment Justin experienced actually added to the adults' fatigue. Understanding that having to deal with his distress was emotionally and physically draining, the consultant acknowledged, "I know a little extra seems like a lot more work, but it sounds like you end up giving it anyway. When Justin clings and cries for a good portion of the morning, you have to attend to his upset and your own." Sue concurred. By the time she arrived, Justin's wailing was replaced by his wreaking havoc on the program. She described the great lengths to which she went to console and control him. Her presence earlier in the process would, she suspected, make it much easier on everyone. All agreed that Sue had a "magic" way with Justin. Hoping to identify characteristics of Sue's relationship that others might emulate if they were demystified, the consultant inquired, "What do you think makes Justin respond so well?" Tometrius attributed Sue's success to her possessing "the patience of Job." Paula complimented Sue's stick-to-itiveness, and Latania talked about her "uncanny ability to anticipate what will set him off." Asking more about each attribute, the consultant was able to extract and articulate reasons for Sue's success, "So it sounds like Justin needs to know that his distress won't make somebody disappear and that when he knows what's coming next change isn't so difficult. I wonder how we could apply that understanding in the morning."

Latania imagined she could make a special point of greeting Justin each morning and reminding him of the routine. Tometrius was glad to be freed of the responsibility and agreed to take on Latania's charges and tasks so her coworker was free to attend to Justin. Mrs. Jones would try to spend a few minutes helping Justin get settled into the program. The consultant wondered if Grandma could, despite her uncertainty, assure Justin of her return at day's end. Seeing and wanting to support her staff and Mrs. Jones'

effort, Paula offered to come into the classroom as this plan was being initiated. Acknowledging the director's contribution, the consultant spoke to
the parallel that was being enacted, "Getting off to a good start is not only
important to Justin. Feeling supported will help everyone begin better.
What comes next is likely to go more smoothly too!"

The group believed Justin's entry would be supported by the ideas that
emerged from the discussion. Additionally, it was agreed that the concepts
could be applied throughout the day. Several subsequent staff meetings were
devoted to talk of transitions. From major changes to slight shifts, Justin's
experience was explored and empathic responses considered.

Sue, the provider who routinely put Justin down to rest, looked for ways of
expanding her intuitive understanding of the fear she felt from Justin. In
response to the consultant's queries, Sue surmised that the letting go that
sleep required was scary especially because her shift ended and she was gone
when Justin woke up. Putting Sue's sense into reassuring words, the consultant suggested that Justin might be helped by hearing who would be available when he woke up and by being reminded when he would next see Sue.

The walk to and from the park was also examined. As Justin loved outdoor
activity, it was difficult for the caregivers to grasp why getting there was hard.
The consultant addressed the confusion by returning to the theory they had
developed together: "Justin's so consumed by what he has to give up that
he can't remember what comes next, but that's where your awareness can
help him." The connection between this and other transitions was becoming clearer to Latania who said, "Sort of like naptime. I guess I thought he
wouldn't be so worried when we were going to do something fun, but now
I get it." Reminded that change, not the anchoring activities, was the
source of upset, the group wanted to relay the concept to Justin. Recognizing
the benefit of forecasting what was to come, the providers agreed to anticipate the daily trip by reminding Justin of what he liked to do at the park.
The consultant applauded this idea but added that it only addressed half
of the equation: "Now he'll know what's coming, but how can you help

him feel that what he's letting go of won't be lost forever? "The idea seemed absurd to Tometrius who scoffed, "You mean we've got to tell him the toys aren't going anywhere? That's crazy." Empathizing with her sense of the notion's extremity, the consultant spoke again to Justin's worldview. The object or activity occupying Justin was not the issue, but it was symbolic of the sense of impermanence he struggled with. Repeatedly reinforcing reality was, the consultant proposed, the only way for Justin to gain security and relinquish the behaviors that bothered them. Unconvinced, Tometrius was willing to give it a shot if it might lead to less commotion. However, willingness was not synonymous with sureness. The providers asked for direction. Voicing a reluctant request, Latania asked, "So what do we say?" Knowing words without action would be unsatisfying to Justin and could unwittingly undermine her advice, the consultant gave voice to the underlying message. Words would have to be paired with responses demonstrating the providers' intentions to preserve Justin's pretransition play. He needed to know that letting go in the moment didn't mean losing something or someone forever. The practical permeations of this concept were infinite. The consultant offered examples. Saving an art activity to which Justin could return was an option. Connection with a peer might continue by suggesting that the pair hold hands on the walk to the park. The train set with which Justin played could be set aside on a tray marked with his name, reminding him that it would be there for him after naptime.

Although illustrating possibilities, these recommendations raised new concerns. The equity for other children was questioned. Preserving toys for one meant limited access for the others. A big to-do about Justin's art project would either be unfair or ignite a need in other children. Aware that the providers' apprehension rendered her ideas undoable, the consultant encouraged a discussion about group versus individual needs. Gaining entrance to the children's experience by way of an analogous adult situation, she harkened back to earlier conversations. Reminding the team that they dealt with discord in their first months together, she talked about their individual needs at that time. New to the center, Latania and Tometrius wanted to feel welcomed, and Sue hoped to be unburdened of responsibility. A blanket response wouldn't have resolved these difficulties. Responding specifically to one did not engender a reciprocal wish in the others. The consultant suggested the same was true for children. The absurdity of being treated identically was jokingly bantered about among the providers. The benefit of being seen as an individual with particular needs was transferred to Justin. The meeting ended with an animated discussion about using containers and carpet squares to concretely convey Justin's territory and mark his possessions.

The preconditions for constructing reparative and ameliorative responsiveness are already established and evident in the meeting that opens this segment. An atmosphere of collaboration surrounds Justin and drives the consultative process. A unanimously held vision of his needs forms a sturdy foundation for fashioning responsive action. The aspects of the consultative stance that created such a surround continue to be employed. Having established her nonpartisan position, the consultant can act as a trusted bridge between Mrs. Jones and the providers and between the providers and the center director. Aware that it will be honored, Mrs. Jones directly divulges her subjective experience. The providers respond in kind. Blame is replaced by shared struggle as it was rendered unproductive and unnecessary.

In this segment of Justin's story, the often-mentioned attribute of wondering finds new purpose. If the group's understanding of Justin's needs is the rudder, the consultant's questions propel the process toward right action. Movement is accelerated by the consultant's suggestions. Although her ideas emanate from her expertise in mental health and early development, she does not announce them from this place but contributes them to the mix. She recognizes that the additive impact is more powerful. The providers (and the grandmother) are the active agents. Therefore, their contributions and willingness to embrace the consultant's advice are essential.

Arriving at intervention strategies through mutual exploration ensures that the providers understand why they, and that they can, employ the chosen course of action. Involving the providers in evolving an intervention strategy for Justin affords the greatest possibility of success. If relating with Justin is based on an internalized belief in the importance of their actions and an authentic sense of efficacy and control over how they respond, the understanding will be utilized in an inclusive range of interactions.

When the providers expressed hesitancy or outright opposition to the consultant's suggestions, as they did toward the end, she pauses the process. The consultant seeks to understand the origin of the obstacle. Faced with the frequent lament that tailored interaction is unfair to the group and will propagate need, the consultant turns her attention to the providers' perceptions. The back-and-forth between the subjective experience of the adults and child oscillates through every phase of the consultative process. The consultant knows that the adults must adapt to or be disabused of this notion of equity before further action can be undertaken.

> Walking into Good Days, the consultant spied a masking tape barricade around a block tower structure. A paper flag with Justin's name fluttered from its top. She smiled to herself as she sat waiting for the teachers to assemble for their meeting. Once everyone was present, she shared her pleasure and asked how they were faring, making explicit her expectation that little of Justin's behavior could have changed in the short time since they last met. All the providers were feeling hopeful about their ability to help Justin despite the fact that his behavior had only incrementally improved. Tometrius admitted that her faith waned when fists flew. Everyone's emotional equilibrium was shaken when Justin became aggressive. Sue tried to console herself and her coworkers by adding, "At least it's less often."

> The consultant reminded them of the fear underneath Justin's outbursts. Even as she spoke to motivation, the consultant was attuned to the anger and anguish that arises when one is hit or kicked. She was equally aware of the impotence providers feel when they are unable to protect other children from being hurt. She voiced her thoughts. "When I remind us all that

Justin lashes out when he is scared, I'm not excusing his actions. Everyone needs to feel safe, Justin, all the children, and you."

Tometrius and Latania vigorously nodded in agreement. Sue's experience was slightly different: "I get kinda down on myself. I can see it coming from across the room, but I can't get to him quick enough."

Imagining that several factors, in addition to speed, prevented Sue's ability to intervene, the consultant talked of the competing demands she and the others were always juggling. She then spotlighted Sue's skill in identifying signs that preceded Justin's difficulties. Sue spoke eloquently about the circumstances that sparked Justin's aggression. Encapsulating the identified triggers, the consultant offers, "Sounds like you see some common hot spots. When Justin is approached unexpectedly, he sees it as a possible attack. If he's asked to abruptly give up someone or something, he lashes out to protect it or you from being taken." Sue thought the consultant captured the essence of the dilemma. Although a revelation, the remarks sounded accurate to Tometrius and Latania.

Awareness of the indicators could, the consultant speculated, alert the caregivers to and aid them in averting trouble. She wondered if proactive preparation for situations that could be predicted to result in mayhem would be useful. Explosions occurred routinely in the dramatic play area, at the water table, and during circle time. The consultant first wondered about and then added to the list of common characteristics of these activities. Each required sharing and a modicum of cooperation. All took place in cramped quarters with many participants. Given that Justin was, as yet, unable to share and felt ganged up on in a group, the consultant wondered what accommodations, if any, the providers could make. Limiting the number of children with whom Justin needed to negotiate was Latania's idea. Although this might work for the water table and dramatic play, Tometrius pointed out that circle time has to be attended by all, and she added, "Sooner or later he's got to learn to share. The real world's not gonna give him everything he wants."

Tometrius' opposition offered the consultant an opportunity to express the intended outcomes of the interventions that the group was contemplating: "Unfortunately, I think the real world, Justin's real world, has, so far taught him exactly the opposite. He's convinced he has to fight to get anything he wants. Only as he begins to believe he can have and hold something, or more importantly someone, will he stop hoarding and start sharing. Think about the times you feel most generous. When there is enough to go around is when we usually feel we can afford to give. That's exactly what we're trying to show Justin."

The virtue of the consultant's ideas was not immediately accepted. Over time, as Justin responded favorably to intervention informed by the consultant's sentiment, the providers trusted it and her more. Tometrius started scooping Justin into her lap at circle time. She made sure he got a turn to talk. She was surprised that the protection that she offered extended his ability to wait and curbed his impulse to clobber children who sat close.

The providers became adept at averting disaster in other areas as well. For a time, individual water basins replaced the communal table. Justin's favorite cooking utensils, replicas of those he watched Granny use in preparing his meals, were reserved on a special tray in the dramatic play area, marking that, for the moment, they were his.

The providers found ways to speak to Justin's misperceptions. The consultant helped craft the communication and, more importantly, convinced the providers of the rationale behind her words. Spying another child's innocent approach, they alerted Justin with words like, "Justin, Omar wants to see what you're cooking. He's not going to take the pan away from you. I'm here to keep you and your toys safe."

As the providers persevered, using their understanding of Justin in increasingly wide and wonderful ways, his sense of security grew. His fear faded. He occasionally offered pretend food he had prepared or shared a portion of his teacher's lap. Days were dotted with difficulty, but fewer were full of disaster. Similarly, the staff's relationship with Mrs. Jones flourished. The adults moved ahead in the spirit of collaboration into which they had entered on Justin's behalf. They saw themselves as standing in solidarity in the efforts to nurture Justin's sense of safety and stability.

These outcomes could signal the end of a successful case consultation. No doubt much was accomplished. Justin no longer consumed his providers' attention nor did talk of him take up all of the consultation conversations. However, the consultant's continued presence at the Good Days Child Care Center allowed ongoing contact with the providers, periodic check-ins about Justin, and the ability to intervene as new developments or obstacles arose.

Consultation Beyond the Classroom

The parameters of case consultation are set by the goal of the effort. When the aim of understanding and ameliorating a child's difficulties in child care is reached, or at least reasonably approached, consultation concludes. However, locating the ideal moment to end is not always clear cut. Reasons for continuing or rekindling consultation around an individual child are numerous. Developments in a child-care program, a family's circumstances, or the child reignite concern and the need to continue or revive the consultation. Ongoing involvement in a program provides the best possibility for immediate response because of the consultant's perpetual presence.

Prolonged or periodically renewed attention to a child is one type of extension. However, issues identified in the course of consultation can call for expansion of other sorts. The consultative context and role is stretched to include aspects of advocacy, case management, and clinical treatment. These additions are not automatic. The rational for and implications of shifting one's stance is carefully considered on a case-by-case basis.

Extended Involvement With Parents: Rationale for Continued Involvement

Factors contributing to a child's difficulties in child care often predate and extend beyond the child-care setting. These contributors are often identified in the course of consultation. Parents' wonderings and concerns about their child may be formulated for the first time in discussions with the consultant. Conversely, longstanding worries about a child's development or the nagging but well-known results of relational disruptions and chronic social pressures are revealed.

In addition to promoting insight and disclosure, the consultative relationship often provides parents an experience with a professional they had not known was possible. The essential elements of the consultant's stance are inherent to any mental health intervention with young children and their caregivers. The consultant treats parents with respect. She is empathic and nonjudgmental. Intrapsychic and interpersonal understanding and the constructs of human motivation guide her interactions. The consultant's behavior also communicates her appreciation of the centrality of relationships. She honors the parent–child relationship as the place where knowledge is held and change will occur. She believes that young children benefit most, whether through consultation or treatment, when one understands and attends to the relational context in which they are developing. This clinical understanding informs the consultation and helps parents elaborate upon and deepen their appreciation of their child's needs.

The continuity between consultation and other forms of mental health intervention are clear. Parents may not articulate the connections as they are stated here, but they feel them. The experience with the consultant is often the impetus for a parent to see the need for and embrace the possibility of additional assistance for their child or themselves. The already established trust in the consultant suggests her as prime candidate to assist. While maintaining a therapeutic stance, the consultant does not have, by virtue of her role, permission to engage in a treatment relationship. The consultant can respond to the parents' request for additional help. However, she does not abandon her consultative posture to do so. Therefore, several factors are considered in determining how to proceed.

The type, intensity, and focus of intervention and the families' resources are considered when contemplating ongoing involvement. Furthering the endeavor of enhancing the child's experience remains central. Assessment leads in one of two directions. If internal and external resources are limited or the need circumscribed and within the consultant's scope of expertise, continued consultation may be offered. Alternatively, families with the emotional, social, and monetary wherewithal to engage services elsewhere are assisted in doing so. Similarly, referrals are offered when intensive intervention or professional expertise outside of the consultants is called for. In either scenario, the reasons for taking a particular path are discussed explicitly and mutually agreed upon.

Ongoing Consultation With Parents

The intent of ongoing direct contact with parents is to help them deepen their understanding of their child. As understanding evolves, ways of responding effectively to the child's needs are considered. This is accomplished through developmental guidance or interventions aimed at enhancing the parents' repertoire of responses. Similar to her work with the child-care providers, the consultant helps parents translate their burgeoning understanding of the child's behavior or developmental needs into responsive action. The process of evolving responsive action is the same as with child-care providers. The ideas for interaction are distinguished by who is involved in them and where they occur. The consultant incorporates what she knows about the child with the particular child-rearing beliefs, cultural values, life circumstances, and capacities of the parent. Together, they come up with a plan for and possible ways of enhancing interaction. Her proposals and strategies are directed at the parent–child relationship as it unfolds and occurs within a family's home life.

Locating or Securing Additional Resources

Children with complex constitutional conundrums, extreme social–emotional disturbances, or severe developmental delays need additional intervention. Children in less profound, but nonetheless problematic predicaments, may also benefit from adjunct services.

At times, providers or parents identify the need for supplemental services prior to the consultant's involvement. However, the need is most often uncovered in the course of consultation. The parents, providers, or both have an inkling that something is amiss. Through the process of consultation, the nature and scope of the concern is clarified. This process is often arduous and occasionally quite painful for parents. The consultant's compassion in unmasking difficulties or disabilities smoothes the path slightly. Reassurance that the consultant will not abandon the parents at the point of a disturbing discovery can also be a comfort.

When exploration reveals a need for additional intervention, the consultant offers to identify referrals for services. The parents' established trust in the consultant increases their willingness to pursue referrals. Parents' suspicions of being scrutinized and judged are relieved. Those who worried that their child would be labeled and left to flounder have had an alternate experience. Having an experience that disconfirms these expectations heightens the parents' belief that another such experience with a different professional is possible.

The consultant ensures the family's engagement with appropriate agencies by accompanying them throughout the process. This may mean initiating and shepherding a family through an assessment for entry into special education or early intervention services. The consultant may escort a parent to an initial visit with an occupational or speech therapist or with a psychotherapist whom she identifies as a prospective provider. Walking with a parent in these ways is not always necessary. Sometime it is not warranted or wanted. However, whether literally going with or walking a parent through the process of securing services, the consultant's presence promotes a comfortable transition.

The consultant's participation in securing services also assists the child-care staff. The consultant's acquaintance with the services she procures allows her to act as a liaison between these professionals and the child-care providers. With the parents' permission, the consultant maintains contact with all of the involved professionals. The consultant acts as a conduit of information. This allows for an exchange of expertise and understanding, which informs and enhances the quality of care offered by all of the providers in a child's life.

Consultant as Advocate

Whether with service providers secured by the consultant or others already involved, several systems and many professionals sometimes attend to children who are the focus of case consultation. Connections to social workers, attorneys, public health nurses, pediatricians, and therapists of all types are common. The difficulties that precipitate consultation capture the attention of, or are related to, these professionals. The reasons for interacting with any of these people are varied. Advocacy is rarely the primary purpose and never the exclusive or initial one. Exchange of information and understanding about the child and the professionals' positions in his or her life is paramount.

The move to negotiate or advocate is carefully considered. Before embracing either activity, the consultant assesses if others, closer to the child, could act more effectively. If possible, the consultant supports the parents or center staff to speak on their own and the child's behalf. Instructing those who will ongoingly act as a child's advocate is empowering and ultimately more effective. However, at times, mitigating factors make the consultant's direct involvement necessary and useful.

The most common reasons are familiarity, time, and expertise. A mental health consultant usually has experience with and is therefore knowledgeable about the systems with which families and providers interface. Familiarity with institutions and their procedures and established relationships with allied professionals allows her to navigate more easily within the public health, school district, child protective services, and juvenile court systems. Additionally, collateral contact is an integral aspect of case consultation. Therefore, the consultant preserves time to meet with agencies or professionals in the child and family's life. Developing and maintaining these relationships takes time. The culture and demands of child care rarely permit such extensive involvement.

Hearing and representing many voices is an essential element of the consultative stance. The consultant employs this skill in advocacy. The added aspect is in representing the collective views of the consultees (provider, parent, or both) to an outside individual or system. In order to voice it, the consultant must genuinely support the perspective. Speaking for a concerned chorus permits her to amplify what they and she believe is in the child's best interest. While doing so, she is attentive to the recipient's views even if they are dramatically different. Understanding need not be synonymous with agreement, but in order to address or amend another's view, theirs must be respectfully entertained and directly responded to. As with other role readjustments, advocacy requires a blending, not an abandonment, of the consultative stance. Unlike the traditional definition, a particular point is not argued nor is support lent solely to one side. The consultant pleads a case for communication and compromise between all parties.

Case Example

Over the course of the next few months, several snags occurred, testing the adults' solidarity and Justin's progress. Some of these obstacles were in Justin's life, and others were in the life of the Good Days Child Care Center, but all affected the climate of the center and efforts to assist Justin. The consultant attended to all of these conundrums—both in their direct impact on Justin and in their effect on the program as a whole.

Each situation is briefly described. The particular action undertaken and the immense effort involved in bringing them to fruition are only touched upon. The broad-stroke treatment in this final chapter of Justin's saga is unlike the tone set in earlier sections. Unelaborated recitation is intended to illustrate the borders of the consultant's role and wide range of activity in which she engages along with and outside of the child-care program.

During the next 6 months, Sue separated from her husband, and an acrimonious custody dispute ensued. An episode of physical violence interrupted Latania's euphoria at having connected with a new partner. These incidences influenced each of their abilities to attend to Justin, or to any of the children in the ways they had previously. They cycled between panic, preoccupied distraction, and depressive disregard. The particulars of their plights elicited specific opposing responses to Justin. Fearful of losing her own child, Sue started to doubt the validity of Justin's removal from his mother. She questioned Mrs. Jones' motivations, making statements like, "I always knew she cared more about the money she gets for taking care of that baby than she does about having him. Why else would anybody in their right mind take on that boy and the three others she's got?" Sue's support of Justin and his grandmother diminished markedly, leaving both baffled and again adrift.

Conversely, Latania's sensitivity to the impact of abuse was heightened. The possibility of Justin's return to his mother, the person who allegedly hurt him, outraged her. Latania's anger reignited the extinguished ember of discord with Sue. Tometrius felt caught in the chasm created by the antagonism. The consultant met with each individually. Special time was set aside for Sue and Latania. Although conversations with the consultant helped Sue recognize that her worries of losing her little one were unfounded, the back-up of a pro bono attorney solidified her sense of security (or eased any residual uncertainties). In addition to securing the lawyer for Sue, the consultant scoured the city for domestic violence services for Latania. Until an appropriate and low-fee therapist was found and Latania's attendance in a group was regular, the consultant routinely checked in to inquire about her safety and support her resolve.

The co-workers' simmering antipathy was overtly addressed through talks initiated at the consultant's urging. Trusting the consultant's intentions, each allowed her to voice the other's position. Over time, reciprocal appreciation was realized and the women's working relationship was repaired. Welcoming the respite from dealing with the daily discord, the director, Paula, made sure coverage for these meetings occurred. Throughout, Paula and the consultant spoke regularly. Together they found ways of maintaining the center's equilibrium during this tough time.

Just as these difficulties were ameliorating, Mrs. Jones was suddenly informed by Justin's social worker that he would be moving in with his mother the following week as a place in a residential program for mothers *with their children* had been secured. Aware that another abrupt transition would jeopardize the still tenuous sense of emotional equilibrium the adults had helped Justin establish, the consultant, at Mrs. Jones' request, assisted her in meeting and negotiating with the social worker for a more tempered transition.

In addition to these meetings in which the consultant spoke about Justin's current functioning and the efforts of all the adults to create some stability for him, the consultant assisted in a myriad of ways. She encouraged and accompanied the social worker to observe Justin in child care. Additionally, she assisted the staff; at their request, in writing a letter to the court expressing their grave concerns about an abrupt move for Justin.

The consultant helped Mrs. Jones to convey to the social worker how much of a risk to Justin's emotional well-being an abrupt change in caregivers would pose. The consultant expressed her strong hope that things would work out well for Justin's mother but suggested that if they did not, and Justin once again was asked to absorb the loss of her and to readjust to yet another change, his resiliency would be severely taxed. As a result of these conversations, the social worker was persuaded of the importance of Justin's remaining at the center and maintaining contact with his grandmother. The director of Horizon House, where Justin's mother was to reside, agreed to accept her even though Justin would spend half of the week at Horizon House and half of the week at his grandmother's home.

The Department of Human Services agreed to provide a transportation worker to drive Justin between Horizon House and his child-care center. The caregivers posted Justin's visitation schedule on the classroom wall and helped Justin each day to remember who would be picking him up in the afternoon and where he was to sleep that night. The consultant was instrumental in initiating and ensuring that these things happened.

In the midst of this work, the consultant was responding to the rekindled anxiety the instability engendered in both Justin and his grandmother. In response to her request for "other old ladies on their last nerve" to commiserate with, Mrs. Jones was referred to a support group for grandparents. Justin, his grandmother, and eventually his mother entered treatment with a therapist secured by the consultant. The clinician and consultant, with Mrs. Jones' permission, exchanged relevant information so as to further strengthen the web of supportive relationships in which Justin would remain securely nested.

In this final segment, the consultant's focus shifts slightly. Reminiscent of the opening phase of this case, the consultant directed her attention to impediments to communication. At this juncture, the conflicts among adults threaten the gains Justin and his caregivers had achieved. The child-care center is, like any other system, ever changing. At times, dynamic shifts are due to changes in individual staff members. Life circumstances, both past and present, influence providers' professional perceptions. Reverberations from the providers' personal lives were witnessed in their treatment of Justin. In this context, the consultant attends to the child-care providers' struggles. The consultant explored details of the providers' dilemmas only with permission. This exploration may be beneficial to the providers in their lives outside the center. However, the consultant is primarily interested in understanding how the providers' experiences impact their treatment of children. This link is made explicit. In addition to her direct assistance, the consultant connected the providers with appropriate resources. Their willingness to talk with her about their troubles was likely linked to their having witnessed and experienced the consultant's nonjudgmental and nonpartisan stance.

Acting on the referrals she offered was an outgrowth of their trust that the consultant's useful stance would be replicated by other helping professionals. Matching services to the providers' existing resources ensured that they could take advantage of the help she offered.

The consultant addressed each provider's dilemma and idiosyncratic response to Justin. As these caregivers' personal concerns converged, the consultant also responded to the conflict between them. While interpreting each one's distress to the other, the consultant fostered the possibility for direct communication. Along the way, she sought to engender empathy for each other, for Justin, and for his grandmother. Even when entertaining their opposing ideas, the consultant held the providers' common concern for Justin as the place to find agreement.

Conflicting ideas as to what was best for Justin characterized the final phase of consultation. The social worker's plan for Justin's placement caused further fissures among the adults. The consultant recalibrated her stance in response to this disagreement.

Assessing that Justin's well-being and his caregivers' efforts could be jeopardized, the consultant stepped in. Acting as an advocate, she spoke to what she and the adults who knew him well felt was in his best interest. Words were not all she offered; she assisted the social worker in seeing and learning about Justin and the child-care center's heroic work with him. Many hours were spent arranging transportation and negotiating scheduling. Concrete planning was accompanied by countless conversations to open channels of conversation. Acting as the bridge between the participants, the consultant helped Mrs. Jones and the center staff appreciate the social worker's constraints and intentions. She inserted Justin's mother into the mix by hypothetically postulating her yearnings and struggle. Agonizing at the thought of Justin losing all that he had come to trust, the consultant was not free from opinion. Guided by her beliefs, she did not get detoured from her role of understanding all of the parties' positions and negotiating cooperative compromises where possible.

Creating collaborative connections with agencies outside of the child-care center involved, but were not limited to, those dealing with Justin's placement. In finding services for him, his grandmother, and the two providers, another aspect of the consultant's usefulness is evidenced. Searching for and securing services that complimented but exceeded her role scaffolded the consultation effort. Willingness to engage with the referrals the consultant located is based, in large measure, on the consultees' well-established foundation of trust in her. With the parties having experienced that support was not only available but also beneficial, other avenues of professional assistance could be entertained.

Confidence in the consultant not only afforded entry but also permitted her ongoing access to the adjunct service providers. As the conduit of information in the expanding sphere that she had a hand in creating, the consultant is able to broaden everyone's awareness of Justin. All of those involved on his behalf have an opportunity to learn from and positively influence the others' understanding and treatment of Justin. Positioned as she was at the interface between these integral influences, the consultant can convey and, more importantly, synthesize the collective experience and expertise she has brought to bear, thereby strengthening Justin's stability and sense of safety.

For a child like Justin, this security was reparative, instilling in him a template of human relationships upon which he can rely in the future. Through case consultations such as this one, the web of supportive relationships within a child-care community and between providers, parents, and outside agencies are strengthened. Fortifying each fiber and helping to weave a resilient web was the goal for Justin as it is for any child around whom mental health consultation is provided.

About the Authors

Kadija Johnston, LCSW

Having worked as a clinical social worker in the field of early childhood mental health since 1982, Kadija Johnston is currently the Director of the Infant–Parent Program at the University of California, San Francisco. She began her career as the coordinator of a therapeutic nursery school and has worked as an infant–parent psychotherapist and consultant to child care. Ms. Johnston has coordinated the Infant–Parent Program's Daycare Consultants since its inception in 1988, which has trained mental health professional in the provision of early childhood mental health services in childcare for over 10 years. Training efforts now extend to consultation programs throughout California. The Program's specialized approach to consultation to childcare has served as a model for other organizations across the country. Ms. Johnston writes and presents widely on early childhood mental health and child-care issues.

Charles Brinamen, PsyD

Dr. Charles Brinamen is a licensed clinical psychologist who supervises and trains interns at Daycare Consultants, a component of the Infant–Parent Program at the University of California, San Francisco. He has been providing mental health consultation to child-care programs in the San Francisco Bay Area for over 10 years and has worked many more years in children's services. He writes and presents nationally on young children, parenting, and child-care consultation. In addition to his work at UCSF, Dr. Brinamen consults to the Visitacion Valley Community Children's Center's therapeutic nursery school, the first of its kind in San Francisco, of which he was a founding member; supervises clinicians; and maintains a private practice. Before joining UCSF in 2002, Dr. Brinamen managed the Children's Council of San Francisco's clinical programs which provide consultation and therapeutic services to children, their families, and their child-care providers. He completed his post-doctoral training at the Infant–Parent Program.